Wicke · Atlas of Radiologic Anatomy

Atlas
of Radiologic Anatomy

Lothar Wicke

With the Collaboration of
Wilhelm Firbas and Roland Schmiedl

Translated and Edited by Anna N. Taylor

Radiographs by
Heinrich Brenner, Wilfried Czech, Erich Deimer, Hans Heeger, Walter Hruby,
Wolfgang Koos, Ernst Kotscher, Emanuele Maranta, Friedrich Olbert,
Axel Perneczky, Peter Probst, Wolfgang Schwägerl, Christl Wicke,
Lothar Wicke and Georg Wolf

Line Drawings by Gabriela Bauer

Fourth English Edition

Urban & Schwarzenberg · Munich–Baltimore 1987

Urban & Schwarzenberg
Pettenkoferstrasse 18
D-8000 Munich 2
Germany

Urban & Schwarzenberg. Inc.
7 East Redwood Street
Baltimore, Maryland 21202
U.S.A.

Address of author:
Lothar Wicke, M.D., Director, Radiologic Institute, Rudolfiner Hospital,
Billrothstraße 78, A-1190 Vienna, Austria

Address of the English translator and editor:
Anna N. Taylor, Ph.D., Professor, Department of Anatomy,
UCLA School of Medicine, Los Angeles, California 90024, U.S.A.

A translation of Atlas der Röntgenanatomie, 3. Auflage, Urban & Schwarzenberg, Munich 1985

Deutsche Bibliothek Cataloguing-in-Publication Data

Wicke, Lothar:
Atlas of radiologic anatomy / Lothar Wicke. With
the collab. of Wilhelm Firbas and Roland Schmiedl.
Transl. and ed. by Anna N. Taylor. Radiographs by
Heinrich Brenner ... Line drawings by Gabriela
Bauer. – 4. Engl. ed. – Munich ; Baltimore :
Urban and Schwarzenberg, 1987.
    Dt. Ausg. u.d.T.: Wicke, Lothar: Atlas der
Röntgenanatomie
    ISBN 3-541-72114-6 (Munich) Kunststoff;
    ISBN 0-8067-2114-6 (Baltimore) Kunststoff

Printed in Germany

ISBN 3-541-72114-6 Munich
ISBN 0-8067-2114-6 Baltimore

Preface to the Fourth English Edition

Unlike translations of earlier editions, this English version of the third German edition translates the entire German text including its historical and technical introduction, discussion of diagnostic imaging techniques, and glossary. The addition of these sections should greatly enhance the utility of this atlas as a reference book for students of radiology. Further, I have tried to maintain the terminology of the labels in conformity with that developed by my esteemed colleague, Dr. Carmine D. Clemente, Professor of Anatomy at the University of California at Los Angeles, in the second edition of his atlas, *Anatomy* (Urban & Schwarzenberg).

I extend special thanks to Dr. James D. Collins, Associate Professor of Radiological Sciences at the UCLA School of Medicine, who reviewed the manuscript for its adherence to current American radiologic usage. I am also grateful to Mr. Braxton D. Mitchell, President of Urban & Schwarzenberg, Baltimore, for giving me the opportunity to work on this project and to his editor, Ms. Starr Belsky, for her numerous constructive suggestions and excellent editorial assistance. I also wish to thank my husband, Kenneth C. Taylor, for his contributions to the translation.

Los Angeles, California, July 1986

Anna Newman Taylor, Ph.D.

Preface to the Third German Edition

Having received numerous requests to reproduce the radiographs as negatives and knowing of improved techniques for producing negative prints, we decided to present the radiographs as they would appear when placed in the viewing box. The publisher generously encouraged this change.

Since publication of the first edition there have been great advances in radiologic imaging techniques. Within the framework of diagnostic imaging, ultrasonography and computed tomography can no longer be neglected. Similarly, MR (Magnetic Resonance Imaging = Nuclear Magnetic Resonance) has advanced from the developmental phase to practical application. In this volume we have included those CT* and MR** images that appeared most important to us, knowing full well that this is only a representative selection from our film library. We trust these images will be an inducement for further study of modern anatomic imaging techniques and lead to an understanding of topographic and cross-sectional anatomy. In order not to exceed the bounds of radiologic anatomy, we have omitted the complex field of ultrasonography. Accordingly, no ultrasonographic images have been included in this edition. We are grateful for the numerous suggestions we received and have tried to implement them wherever and whenever possible.

We thank the publishers for their generosity and support in the production of this revised edition.

Vienna, September 1985

Lothar Wicke, M.D., F.I.C.A.

Wilhelm Firbas, M.D.

Roland Schmiedl, M.D.

---

* The CT images were made with a Toshiba TCT 80A.

** We thank the Odelga Company (distributors of Technicare products in Austria) for allowing us to use Technicare's MR images.

Preface to the First German Edition

The ever-increasing inclusion of radiologic diagnosis in anatomic instruction and clinical training has prompted the organization of this volume. It affords students an opportunity to check and expand their knowledge of the anatomic details observable by radiology, with guidance from the drawings accompanying each radiograph.

The illustrations have been selected to give the broadest possible basic coverage of radiologic anatomy. In our opinion they include the most common radiologic examinations with which students, technicians, and house staff may be confronted. We have intentionally dispensed with many specialized exposure and projection techniques that would have exceeded the intended scope of the book and that are readily accessible in more specialized works. In order to retain the character of the atlas we have kept the textual portion as short as possible. The major part of the information contained herein concerning contrast media, figures, and technical drawings was generously provided by the Schering and Siemens Companies. Clarification of all other technical details and description of experimental findings is, in our opinion, the task of clinical radiology using "radiologic anatomy" as its basis.

We are indebted to our professor of anatomy, Dr. W. Krause, for his generous and critical supervision of the captions and labeling of the illustrations in the atlas. We are also grateful to the publishers for their care in achieving optimal reproduction of the radiographs and line drawings. The original radiographs were electronically contrast-enhanced and converted into positives for use in the book, since only in this form do we feel the best detail is to be captured. The disadvantage, namely that the radiographs do not appear as negatives, the way radiologists see them in practice, is outweighed in our opinion by the picture quality. As for terminology, we used the Wiesbaden anatomic nomenclature of 1965, as often as suitable terms were available. Special designations that are only in clinical or radiologic use are marked with an asterisk (*).

It is our hope that, with this atlas, we have made available a practical ready-reference guide for those interested in acquiring a basic knowledge of radiologic anatomy as applied to clinical radiology.

Vienna, December 1976

Lothar Wicke, M.D., F.I.C.A.

Wilhelm Firbas, M.D.

Roland Schmiedl, M.D.

Table of Contents

Prefaces V

Introduction X

History X
Physical units in diagnostic radiology XI
Properties of x-radiation XI
Radiographic equipment XI
Fluoroscopic and x-ray television equipment . . . XIII

Diagnostic Imaging Techniques XV

Plain films XV
Negative contrast media XV
Positive contrast media XVI

ATLAS 1

Skull

Skull (p.a., lateral, axial) 2
Skull, computed tomography (axial series) 10
Paranasal sinuses (p.a., inclined, half axial) 16
Orbits (p.a.) 18
Optic canal (Rhese) 20
Temporal bone (semisagittal, Stenvers; half
lateral, Schuller; half axial, Mayer) 20
Petrous bone, computed tomography (axial,
pneumocisternography) 24
Upper and lower jaws (panoramic) 26
Carotid angiography (lateral, a.p., venous phase) 28
Vertebral angiography (lateral, a.p., venous phase) 40
Ventriculography (a.p., lateral, Pantopaque) . . . 46
Sella turcica (coned-down image) 50
Brain, computed tomography (axial series) 52
Magnetic resonance imaging (axial, parasagittal) 58

Vertebral Column

Cervical spine (a.p., dens of axis a.p.) 62
Atlantoaxial joint, computed tomography (axial) 66

Cervical spine (lateral, flexion, extension,
oblique) 68
Cervical spine, myelography (p.a.) 76
Thoracic spine (a.p., lateral, oblique) 78
Thoracic spine, computed tomography (axial
series of T4–T5) 82
Lumbar spine (a.p., lateral, oblique) 84
Lumbar spine, myelography (p.a., oblique,
lateral) 90
Lumbar spine, computed tomography (axial
series of L4/L5) 96

Pelvis

Pelvis (a.p.) 102
Sacrum and coccyx (lateral) 104
Pelvic arteries, angiography 106

Upper Extremity

Shoulder (a.p., axial) 108
Elbow (a.p., lateral) 112
Elbow, angiography 114
Hand (dorsovolar, lateral, lateral oblique) 116
Hand, angiography 122

Lower Extremity

Hip joint (a.p., leg laterally abducted, child's) . . 124
Knee joint (a.p., lateral) 130
Knee joint, arthrography (lateral,
patella axial, a.p.) 134
Knee joint, angiography (a.p.) 138
Ankle joint (a.p., lateral, oblique) 140
Foot (dorsoplantar, lateral) 144
Foot, angiography (a.p.) 148

Thorax and Neck

Lungs (p.a., lateral) 150
Lungs, tomography (a.p.) 154

Bronchography (right: a.p., slight oblique; left: a.p., slight oblique) 156
Mediastinography (lateral tomogram) 164
Heart (p.a., right anterior oblique, left anterior oblique) 166
Heart, angiocardiography (right and left ventricles) 172
Heart, digital subtraction angiography 176
Heart, magnetic resonance imaging (frontal, sagittal, transverse) 178
Aortic arch, angiography 180
Coronary angiography (right: left anterior oblique, lateral; left: right and left anterior oblique) 184
Mammography (craniocaudal, lateral) 192
Trachea (p.a., lateral) 196

Digestive Tract

Hypopharynx (deglutition: p.a., lateral) 200
Esophagus (right anterior oblique, p.a.) 204
Stomach (p.a. upright, p.a. supine) 208
Stomach, fundus (coned-down images: a.p. prone, p.a. upright) 214
Stomach, pylorus, and duodenal bulb (coned-down p.a. supine) 216
Small intestine 218
Celiac angiography 220
Splenoportography 222
Superior mesenteric artery, angiography 224
Inferior mesenteric artery, angiography 226
Upper abdomen, computed tomography (axial sections) 228
Large intestine (barium enema, lateral; double contrast) 232

Gall Bladder and Biliary Ducts

Gall bladder, oral cholecystography (after ingestion and contraction) 236

Biliary ducts, intravenous cholangiography 240
Biliary ducts, retrograde cholangiography 242
Biliary ducts, intraoperative cholangiography . . . 244

Kidneys and Urinary Tract

Kidneys and urinary tract, intravenous urography 246
Kidneys and urinary tract, intravenous urography (section of left kidney) 248
Selective renal angiography 248
Abdominal aortography 250
Pneumoretroperitoneal tomography 252
Adrenal glands, computed tomography (axial) . . 254

Veins

Left lower extremity, venography (a.p., lateral) . . 256
Venous valve, venography 258

Lymphatics

Pelvic lymphography (a.p.) 260
Abdominal lymphography (a.p., lateral) 262
Pelvic and abdominal lymphography (oblique) . . 266
Inguinal lymphography 268
Axillary lymphography 270
Thoracic duct, lymphography 272

Gynecologic Radiography

Hysterosalpingography 274
Fetography 276

Glossary 279

Bibliography 281

Subject Index 282

Introduction

History

On November 8, 1895, thirty-six years after the discovery of cathode rays and two years after the development of the Lenard tube (cathode ray tube), William Conrad Roentgen discovered "a new kind of ray," which he termed an x-ray. The first medical radiograph was made only a few days later, on December 22, by Roentgen and was reported in a preliminary paper that he submitted for publication on December 28. The medical profession reacted very quickly. On January 6, 1896, the Berlin Society for Internal Medicine called a meeting. One lecture topic was "Roentgen's experiments with cathode rays and their diagnostic application," which stated, in part: "This is particularly important for medicine. Certainly, surgery should derive advantage from photographs of bone *in vivo*. Fractures, dislocations, swellings, foreign bodies should be easily recognizable; I also call attention to the sharp outlines of the lucent interphalangeal joints which are apparent on the radiographs, making joint margins visible. It is also possible that various changes will be recognizable within the body cavity, since the rays outline the visceral margins and make visible such conditions as dense tumors, obstructive intestinal disease, fecal impaction."

Daily newspapers, foremost of which were *The Press*, whose publishers correctly recognized the significance of the discovery for medicine, the *Frankfurter Zeitung*, and the *Vossische Zeitung* reported Roentgen's discovery. On January 13, 1896, the first report appeared in a medical journal, the *Berliner Klinische Wochenschrift*. Worldwide development of the field of diagnostic radiology then began (Fig. 1). In 1896, there appeared over 1000 publications regarding the new imaging technique. Journals appeared, such as *Archives of the Roentgen Ray (Archives of Clinical Skiagraphy)*, *American X-Ray Journal*, and *Fortschritte auf dem Gebiet der Röntgenstrahlen (Advances in the Field of X-Rays)*. Institutes of Radiology were founded in Hamburg, Berlin, London, Boston, and New York. Of the pioneers in this field, many of whom became victims of their own experimentation, only a few can be mentioned here: Albers-Schönberg (1919, first professor of roentgenology in Germany); Levy-Dorn (stereoscopic radiographs, 1897); Zuppinger (alterations of the skeletal system); Gocht (first postoperative reference radiographs); Grashey (use of an x-ray apparatus on the operating table, 1904); Köhler ("Boundaries of Normal and Incipient Pathology on Radiographs," 1905); Rieder (application of contrast medium in the examination of the gastrointestinal tract, 1904); Holzknecht (lungs, diaphragm, etc., 1901; investi-

gations of abdominal tumors, 1906); Haudek (Haudek's niche, 1910); Chaoul and dall'Acqua (normal and pathologic anatomy of the digestive tract); Åkerlund (diagnosis of duodenal ulcers and hiatal hernias); Béclère (tuberculosis); Pancoast and Pendergrass (lung alterations in dust inhalation); Stewart, Sicard, and Forestier (bronchography); Bocage and Vallebona (tomography, 1922 and 1930); Janker (cineradiography); Forssmann, Voelker, and Lichtenberg; Roseno and Swick; Graham and Cole; Heuser; Dandy; Dos Santos; Hoffa; Lorey; and Ruiz-Rivas, among many others.

The field of radiation therapy developed almost simultaneously with diagnostic radiology (irradiation of a heavily pigmented hairy nevus by Freund in Vienna, the first successful treatment of skin cancer, 1899). In 1901, W. C. Roentgen received the first Nobel Prize in physics for his discovery of x-rays. Obviously, x-rays are thus essential to both diagnosis and therapy in current medical practice.

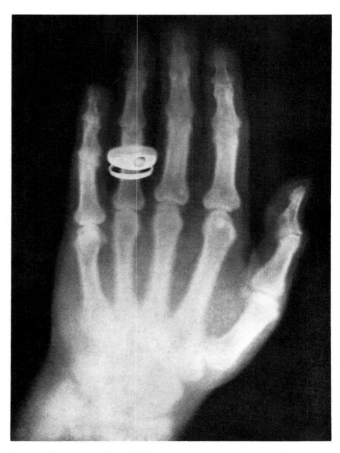

Fig. 1. The hand of Dr. Kölliker, anatomist, photographed by Roentgen on January 23, 1896.

In Vienna long-standing ties exist between clinical diagnostic radiology (Holzknecht, Schüller, E. G. Mayer) and radiographic anatomy (Goldhamer). Radiographic anatomy forms a bridge between the pre-clinical studies and the clinical subspecialities; it teaches students to systematically apply their knowledge of gross anatomy in the interpretation of radiographic images. Gross anatomy consists primarily of a three-dimensional approach to color-differentiated preparations and models of the human body, whereas radiologic anatomy teaches students to correlate the gross anatomic structures with the density variations of two-dimensional images. Special diagnostic procedures must be mastered in order to discern the individual organs and structures within the human body.

Physical Units in Diagnostic Radiology

In 1969, the General Conference on Weights and Measures formulated the International Unit System (Système Internationale des Unités, SI) based upon the seven fundamental units: meter (m), kilogram (kg), second (s), ampere (A), kelvin (K), mole (mol), and candela (cd). All other units in the decimal system are obtainable via multiplication or division and are expressible as derived units.

Since the old units are still current in radiology, they are listed below in terms of SI units.

Units of Energy:

1 eV (electron volt): A particle having a charge of one electron (e) has a kinetic energy of 1 eV after passing through a potential difference of 1 volt (V) in a vacuum.

1 keV (thousand electron volts) = 10^3 eV
1 MeV (million electron volts) = 10^6 eV

Ionizing Radiation:

The ionizing radiation is determined by the quantity of charge (measured in coulombs, C) produced in a quantity of matter (measured in kilograms). Its unit is the roentgen (R).

1 R = $2.58 \cdot 10^{-4}$ C/kg
SI: coulomb per kilogram
In air, under normal conditions, 1 R produces $2.1 \cdot 10^9$ ion pairs/cm³.

Absorbed Radiation:

The rad (rad) is the unit of absorbed energy [measured in joules (J) per kilogram] per unit of mass.

1 rad = 0.01 J/kg = 100 erg/g
SI: joule per kilogram
1 gray (Gy) = 1 J/kg

Properties of X-Radiation

X-rays are electromagnetic waves that have the properties of penetrating matter, exposing films, and exciting fluorescent material. In penetrating matter, x-rays may transfer energy in several ways: classical scattering, the Compton effect, the photoelectric effect, and absorption. The properties as described are used in diagnostic radiology (radiography and fluoroscopy).

Radiographic Equipment

In modern practice, six-pulse generators (Fig. 2), which guarantee a fairly constant level of current, are used almost exclusively. Special procedures, such as angiocardiography, use high-powered twelve-pulse generators. The focal spot of the rotating anode tube does not exceed 0.3 mm × 0.3 mm in size. Smaller focal spots (0.1 mm × 0.1 mm) are recommended for specific cases, such as bone structure analysis or angiography, where it is necessary to produce enlarged images. To

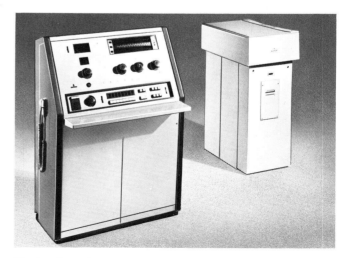

Fig. 2. Control console and six-pulse generator.

obtain the highest image quality, the irradiated volume should be kept as small as possible. Stray radiation can be kept to a minimum by limiting the field by means of lead collimators.

Since x-rays diverge conically from the anode of the x-ray tube, the magnification and sharpness of an image will depend upon the target and film distances. The smallest possible target-film distance and the largest possible target-focus or film-focus distance are usually chosen.

X-ray films are contained in a film cassette that has an intensifier screen on either side of the film. When the x-ray passes through the cassette, the intensifier screens fluoresce and expose the film. The intensification of the screens ranges from low (slight darkening) to relatively high intensification, the latter resulting in loss of sharpness.

For difficult cases and for relatively thin objects (hands, feet), cassetteless radiography has been used; however, film-screen combinations should be considered, depending upon the information desired. Cassetteless radiography has the advantage of good signal definition (through elimination of screen artefacts) but has the disadvantage of requiring a higher dosage.

A grid is used to avoid unnecessary scattered radiation when examining dense objects (e.g., chest, abdomen, pelvis). The grid may be placed in the cassette between the object and the front screen, or, more frequently, in the radiographic table or in the cassette holder (Fig. 3) as a moving grid between the target and cassette (Bucky-Potter diaphragm) (Fig. 4). The slits in the grid are centered at the focus of the tube and thereby allow only

radiation that has been attenuated by absorption in various degrees to pass through to the film-screen combination. The rapid movement of the Bucky diaphragm eliminates grid lines.

Blurring due to grid motion is used to advantage in tomography. In this technique the x-ray tube and cassette move in opposite directions, either linearly, circularly,

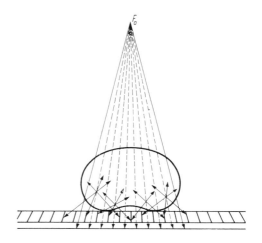

Fig. 4.   Method of operation of a focusing grid.

elliptically, or hypocycloidally about a fulcrum within the target (Fig. 5). Usually, by raising or lowering the examination table, the fulcrum (sectional plane) is changed with respect to the object, and this changes the cross-sectional plane under examination. By virtue of the oscillation of the x-ray tube and film plane around a fulcrum, only structures in the plane of the fulcrum are sharply defined; other structures lying above or below

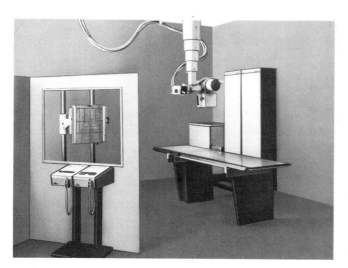

Fig. 3.   Radiographic table, cassette holder (left); switching element and electrical cabinet with power divider (right).

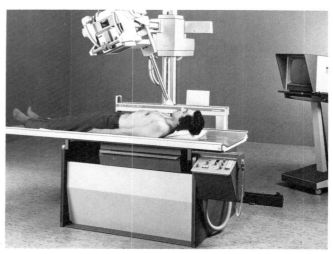

Fig. 5.   Radiographic and scanning equipment with floating table.

the plane are diffuse (Fig. 6). In tomography, sections of 1 cm to 1 mm, depending upon the form of movement, can be examined. When the tomographic angle is small, i.e., in zonography, the thickness of the section is large (several centimeters) and sharply defined (used for kidney, gall bladder, or biliary ducts). The technique of

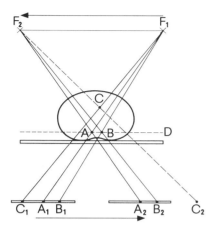

Fig. 6. Schematic representation of longitudinal geometric tomography.

transverse axial tomography, in which the tube remains fixed and the patient as well as the film cassette is rotated about the same axis, is no longer in general use but has now experienced a revival in interest through computed tomography. In the latter technique, a tube and films situated opposite the x-ray tube are rotated around the supine subject. The x-rays are differentially attenuated and impinge on the films. This attenuation is measured at various angles, its magnitude being transmitted to a

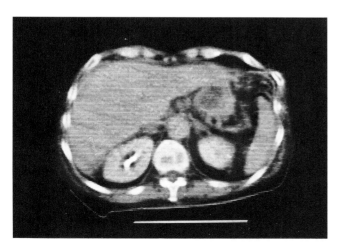

Fig. 7. Computed tomograph (cross-sectional cut) of upper abdominal organs [liver, kidneys (right with contrast medium), aorta, diaphragm, spleen].

computer that can generate gray values corresponding to absorption levels (Fig. 7) or produce a color picture on a monitor.

If one wishes to observe the various filling phases of the heart or vessels by using a contrast medium, this may be done directly with a sheet film changer or indirectly with small film (35 mm, 70 mm, 100 mm) and the aid of a film intensifier.

Special equipment has been developed for certain techniques, such as tomography and radiography, mammography, and skeletal imaging.

Fluoroscopic and X-Ray Television Equipment

The movements of different organs (e.g., heart, diaphragm, gastrointestinal tract) may be studied by means of fluoroscopy. In the early days of radiology, zinc cadmium sulfide was used in fluorescent screens.[*] These have now been largely replaced by the image-intensifier television monitoring system. In this system the x-rays impinge on the input screen of an image-intensifier tube and produce an electron image on the photocathode. These photoelectrons, after being accelerated and focused by an electron lens system, strike the output screen, producing an image that is smaller but

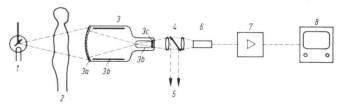

Fig. 8. 1. X-ray tube; 2. patient; 3. image intensifier; 3a. photocathode; 3b. electron lens; 3c. phosphor screen; 4. tandem optics; 5. cable to motion picture camera; 6. television camera; 7. intensifier; 8. television monitor.

10,000 times brighter than the image at the input screen (Fig. 8). This can be either viewed directly (in rare cases) or relayed to a television monitor via an attached television camera and electronic image intensifier. In contrast to older techniques, the image-intensifier television system has the advantage of greater resolution along with

---

[*] The fluorescent screen produces an image, and its brightness is solely dependent upon the intensity of radiation falling upon it.

Introduction

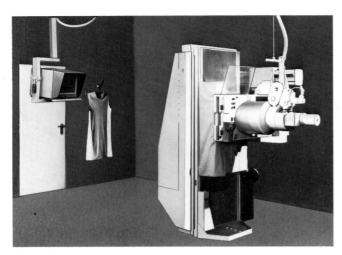

Fig. 9. Modern fluoroscopic apparatus with image-intensifier television system.

reduced radiation exposure for patients, technicians, and physicians, especially when an automatic dose regulator is available.* Modern fluoroscopic equipment (Fig. 9) can store relevant information on film or record the movement of organs on cinefilm or magnetic tape. The image intensifier coupled with the television monitor reduces radiation dosage by about half compared to the fluorescent screen technique; use of the image-intensifier camera reduces radiation by about 90% compared with conventional cassette techniques. Some medical specialties, such as neurosurgery and urology, have their own special techniques and require customized fluoroscopic equipment.

Summary

A. X-Ray Photography

1. Direct

    a) Cassetteless photography (film packed in light-tight containers)

    b) Cassette photography (film sealed in light-tight aluminum or plastic cassettes between two intensifier screens)

       1) Without Bucky diaphragm

       2) With Bucky diaphragm

    c) Sheet-film changer (changer for angiography)

2. Indirect

    a) Photography using image intensifiers

       1) Still photography (70 mm, 100 mm)

       2) Cinematography (35 mm)

    b) Photography using a television system

       1) With special camera from the television monitor (rather seldom)

       2) Video tape recording (VTR) on magnetic tape

3. Special Procedures

    a) Xeroradiography**

    b) Computed tomography (CT)

B. X-Ray Fluoroscopy

1. Fluorescent screen – almost obsolete
2. Image-intensifier television fluoroscopy

---

* Control of dose rate up to specified values by automatic exposure devices. This results in consistent picture quality independent of patient density, along with reduction of radiation exposure.

** Radiological photographic dry-imaging method using electrostatic images and special development techniques.

Diagnostic Imaging Techniques

Plain Films

Plain films are routine radiographs made directly, without resorting to any use of contrast material, and therefore are solely produced by differential beam absorption in various organs. The absorption is dependent upon the tissue density (grams per cubic centimeter). Bones have an approximate density of 1.9 and produce a "skeletal dense" shadow on the x-ray image; this appears dark on a fluoroscopic image and light on a plain film (negative). Soft tissues (e.g., muscle, cartilage, fat, blood) have a density of 1.0, so that x-rays are fairly evenly absorbed, producing a grayish "soft tissue compactness" in the fluoroscopic image and on the film. Air has the lowest density (0.0013), producing a light area on the picture screen and a darkening (transparency in radiologic terminology) on the negative film (e.g., lung, tracheal lumen, paranasal sinuses, intestinal gas) (Fig. 10).

An additional factor contributing to attenuation of the primary beam is dispersion (see discussion under "Radiographic Equipment"). Thus the x-ray finally emerging from the body is reduced in intensity by absorption and dispersion. On the plain film, attenuation effects (absorption and dispersion) through various tissues are distinguished as

1. air-containing structures (slight attenuation), e.g., lung;
2. soft tissue density (moderate attenuation), e.g., breast;
3. skeletal density (greater attenuation).

Dental fillings or positive contrast media can be identified on plain films by virtue of their high density.

In order to overcome the absence of differences in attenuation within soft tissues (gall bladder, kidney, liver, vessels, and so forth), various kinds of contrast media are administered.

Negative Contrast Media

Negative contrast media are gaseous substances that enhance the contrast between the various soft tissues.

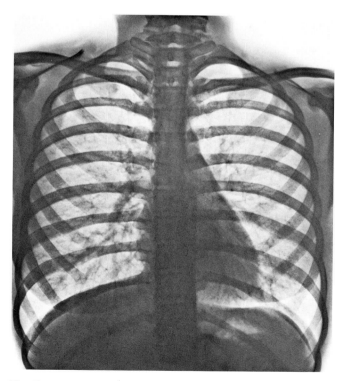

Fig. 10a. Fluoroscopy of thorax (or positive copy). Radiolucent structures appear as lighter areas (lungs, trachea, fundus of stomach); radiopaque structures appear as organ densities (bones, heart).

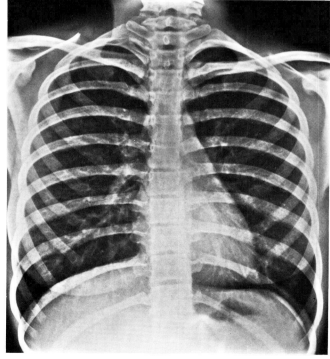

Fig. 10b. Gray-value reproduction of an original x-ray film (photographic negative). The dark areas (radiolucent) correspond to the light or transparent regions of Fig. 10a (trachea, lungs, fundus of stomach), whereas regions that are white or gray on the film correspond to the organ densities of Fig. 10a (bones, heart, soft tissues).

Thus, for example, in pneumoencephalography, cerebrospinal fluid is siphoned from the ventricles and a gas mixture is insufflated, so that the now air-containing ventricle is contrasted by becoming more radiolucent than the surrounding cerebral tissues. In pneumoperitoneal studies (see Fig. 151), about 1000 ml of gas are insufflated presacrally, with the patient in the prone position; the gas rises slowly in the connective tissues of the retroperitoneal cavity to surround the kidneys and adrenals and differentiate them from the surrounding muscular portions. The principle of mediastinography (see Fig. 106) is similar. The use of gases in pneumoperitoneal studies and in mediastinography has now been superceded by ultrasound, computed axial tomography, magnetic resonance imaging, and tomography, as well as by isotopic procedures. Gases used for negative contrast include air, oxygen, nitrogen, nitrous oxide, and carbon dioxide. Positive and negative contrast media can be used in combination to produce the double-contrast method, which is employed for difficult diagnoses of the gastrointestinal tract (see Fig. 141, Gastrovision with barium sulfate) or in arthrography (see Figs. 89 and 91).

Positive Contrast Media

Positive contrast materials absorb x-rays more intensely than soft tissue or bone. Because of their higher density and advantageous chemical properties, two substances have proven particularly useful for radiologic diagnosis: barium and iodine compounds.

Water-Insoluble Contrast Media:

Barium sulfate ($BaSO_4$) is used as a suspension in various consistencies (normal barium suspension, barium relief, barium paste). It is the material of choice for radiologic diagnosis of the gastrointestinal tract. There is an increasing availability of commercial products containing flavored additives and various mucosal adhesive materials (e.g., Barosperse, barium with CO_2).

Oily Contrast Media:

Oily contrast media consist of iodized oils. Since they are not resorbed and additionally produce fat embolism, their indication is very circumscribed and primarily limited to lymphography (Ethiodol), representation of the brain ventricles, myelography, and computed tomography (Omnipaque). After withdrawal of cerebrospinal fluid, the radiopaque contrast medium is introduced into the fluid space and is withdrawn after termination of the examination.

Water-Soluble Contrast Media:

Water-soluble contrast media are sodium or methylglucamine salts of triiodinated benzoic acid. They either are administered orally and then absorbed from the intestine and excreted through the liver, or are delivered intra-arterially or intravenously and likewise excreted through the liver or kidneys. Increasingly, nonionized contrast media are being used that are both better tolerated and have fewer side effects. On the day before a gall bladder examination, the patient is given a contrast medium orally (e.g., Bilopaque), which is absorbed through the intestinal epithelium, extracted by the liver, and reaches the gall bladder via the biliary ducts; in cholangiography (large bile ducts) and in cholecystangiography (gall bladder), the contrast medium is administered intravenously. In myelography of the lower quadrant (distal spinal cord), a water-soluble contrast medium can likewise be used (e.g., Omnipaque). For representation of the vessels (veins, arteries, cardiac chambers), contrast media of varying concentrations and chemical compositions are commercially available (e.g., Renografin, Conray). Contrast materials are also available for demonstration of the kidneys (Renografin, Conray). Dionosil is used as an agent for bronchography, and Sinografin (aqueous) or Ethiodol is used for hysterosalpingography.

For demonstration of the veins (phlebography or venography), a contrast medium is injected into the veins and radiographs are taken at specified intervals. In the representation of the arterial tree (arteriography), vessels in favorable locations can be punctured directly, and the contrast medium is injected via the puncture needle or administered into the vessel via an advancing catheter (e.g., Seldinger technique). Thus, for example, in exploratory angiography of the abdominal region, selective or sometimes superselective demonstration of an individual vessel can be achieved. The individual filling phases (early arterial, late arterial, parenchymal, venous) are recorded directly either with a film changer or on cine- and video recorders.

For urograms the kidney or the pelvic calyx system of the kidney is represented at specific time intervals. In this technique the intravenous contrast medium (e.g., Renografin) reaches the kidney via the pulmonary circulation, the aorta, and the renal vessels whence it is excreted.

Atlas

The figures in the atlas are reduced pictures of original x-ray films of living persons, except for Fig. 15, which is an axial view of the base of the skull, taken from a skeleton without mandibles.

In roentgenology, directions are specified such that the central ray always passes through the patient from the x-ray tube to the film cassette or screen. X-ray pictures are observed in a corresponding manner, that is, as if the patient were standing in front of the examiner. There are a few exceptions to this rule in practice (e.g., hand dorsal-palmar, foot dorsal-plantar).

Lead markers are frequently placed on an x-ray film in order to identify the respective body half (R for right, L for left). Time markers are added for pictures taken at specified intervals of time after the final injection (e.g., in urograms).

In order to determine an exact localization in the body, radiographs are frequently taken in directions of the beam other than those of sectional roentgenography. Thus, radiographs of the skull are taken in the posterior-anterior and in the lateral (= frontal) x-ray direction; when x-raying the stomach, or especially while taking radiographs during cardiac diagnostics, fluoroscopy is recommended and radiographs should be taken in both oblique projections. The most important directional specifications are listed below (Fig. 11).

(1) p.a.: posterior-anterior (in this case in the median-sagittal plane);
(2) lateral: from the side (right to left, or left to right);
(3) frontal: parallel to the frontal plane;
(4) right anterior oblique projection (the fencer's position): the patient is positioned around his vertical axis such that the x-rays pass through from the left back to the right front;
(5) left anterior oblique projection (the boxer's position): the patient is positioned around his vertical axis so that the x-rays pass through from the right back to the left front;
(6) sagittal: parallel to the median plane (p.a. or a.p.);
(7) tangential: the central ray is tangential to a curved surface at one point;

a.p.: anterior-posterior;
ds: from right (dexter) to left (sinister);
sd: from left (sinister) to right (dexter);
dv: (concerning the hand) = dorsovolar (palmar): from the back of the hand to its palm;
dp: dorsoplantar: from the back of the foot to its sole;
radio-ulnar: from the radius to the ulna;
axial: in the direction of the longitudinal axis of the body when standing upright.

In addition, anatomic specifications such as cranial, caudal, proximal, distal, dorsal, ventral and transversal are valid.

To simplify conceptualization, diagrams are given indicating the manner in which the x-ray films were taken. The central axis of the x-ray beam is marked with an arrow to show its direction and the film cassette is shown by a thick line.

The orbito-meatal line (connecting line between the lower margin of the orbit and the upper border of the external auditory canal) is drawn with a dash-dot-dash line (–·–·–). Special designations that are only in clinical or radiologic use are marked with an asterisk (*).

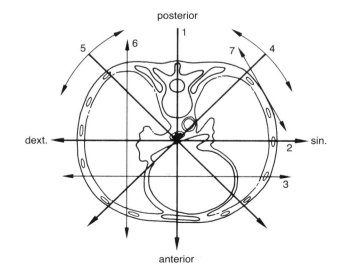

Fig. 11. Frequently used directional markers, as applied to a cross-section of the thorax.

Skull

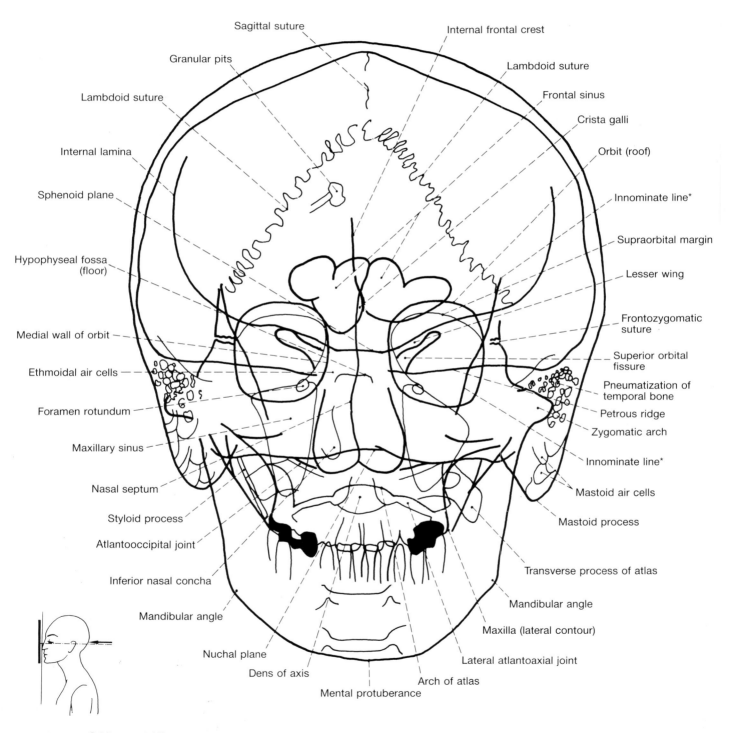

Sagittal suture

Granular pits

Lambdoid suture

Internal lamina

Sphenoid plane

Hypophyseal fossa
(floor)

Medial wall of orbit

Ethmoidal air cells

Foramen rotundum

Maxillary sinus

Nasal septum

Styloid process

Atlantooccipital joint

Inferior nasal concha

Mandibular angle

Nuchal plane

Dens of axis

Mental protuberance

Internal frontal crest

Lambdoid suture

Frontal sinus

Crista galli

Orbit (roof)

Innominate line*

Supraorbital margin

Lesser wing

Frontozygomatic
suture

Superior orbital
fissure

Pneumatization of
temporal bone

Petrous ridge

Zygomatic arch

Innominate line*

Mastoid air cells

Mastoid process

Transverse process of atlas

Mandibular angle

Maxilla (lateral contour)

Lateral atlantoaxial joint

Arch of atlas

·—·—·— = Orbito-meatal line

2

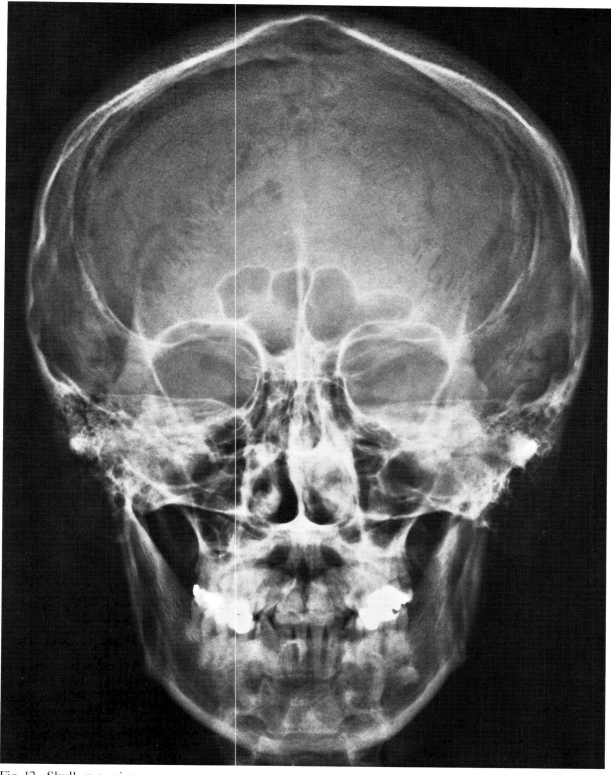

Fig. 12. Skull, p.a. view

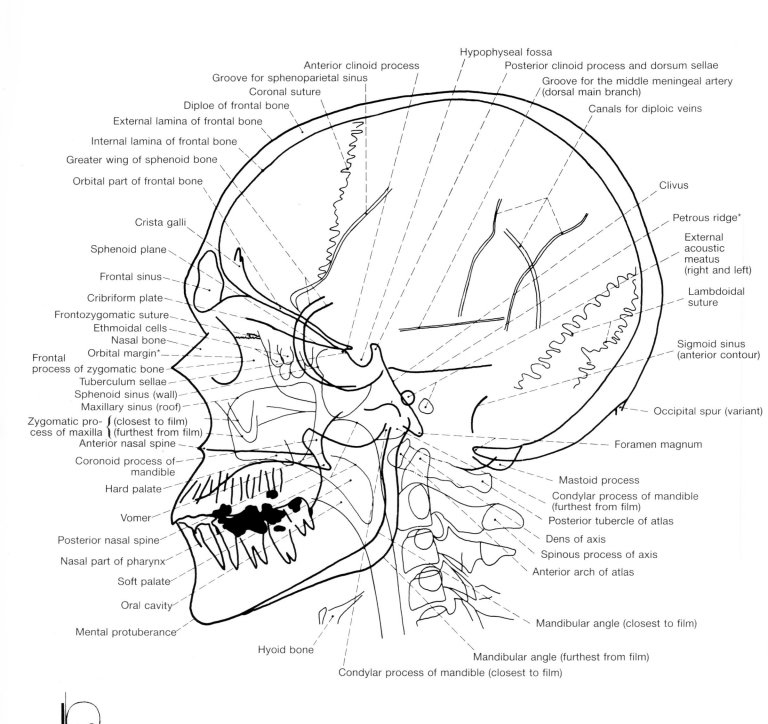

Anterior clinoid process

Hypophyseal fossa

Posterior clinoid process and dorsum sellae

Groove for sphenoparietal sinus

Groove for the middle meningeal artery
(dorsal main branch)

Coronal suture

Diploe of frontal bone

Canals for diploic veins

External lamina of frontal bone

Internal lamina of frontal bone

Greater wing of sphenoid bone

Clivus

Orbital part of frontal bone

Petrous ridge*

Crista galli

External
acoustic
meatus
(right and left)

Sphenoid plane

Frontal sinus

Lambdoidal
suture

Cribriform plate

Frontozygomatic suture

Ethmoidal cells

Nasal bone

Sigmoid sinus
(anterior contour)

Frontal
process of zygomatic bone

Orbital margin*

Tuberculum sellae

Sphenoid sinus (wall)

Maxillary sinus (roof)

Occipital spur (variant)

Zygomatic pro- {(closest to film)
cess of maxilla {(furthest from film)

Foramen magnum

Anterior nasal spine

Coronoid process of
mandible

Mastoid process

Hard palate

Condylar process of mandible
(furthest from film)

Vomer

Posterior tubercle of atlas

Posterior nasal spine

Dens of axis

Nasal part of pharynx

Spinous process of axis

Soft palate

Anterior arch of atlas

Oral cavity

Mental protuberance

Mandibular angle (closest to film)

Hyoid bone

Mandibular angle (furthest from film)

Condylar process of mandible (closest to film)

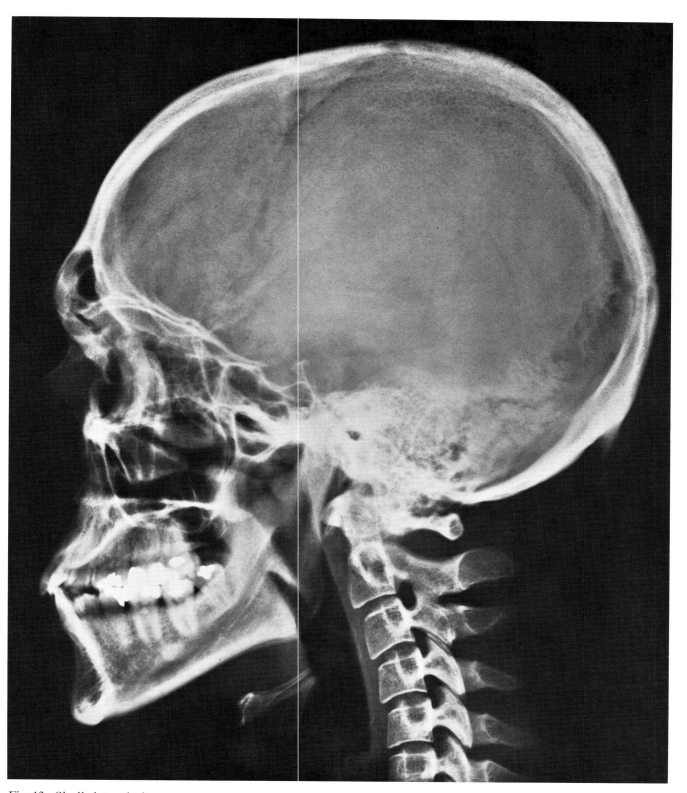

Fig. 13. Skull, lateral view

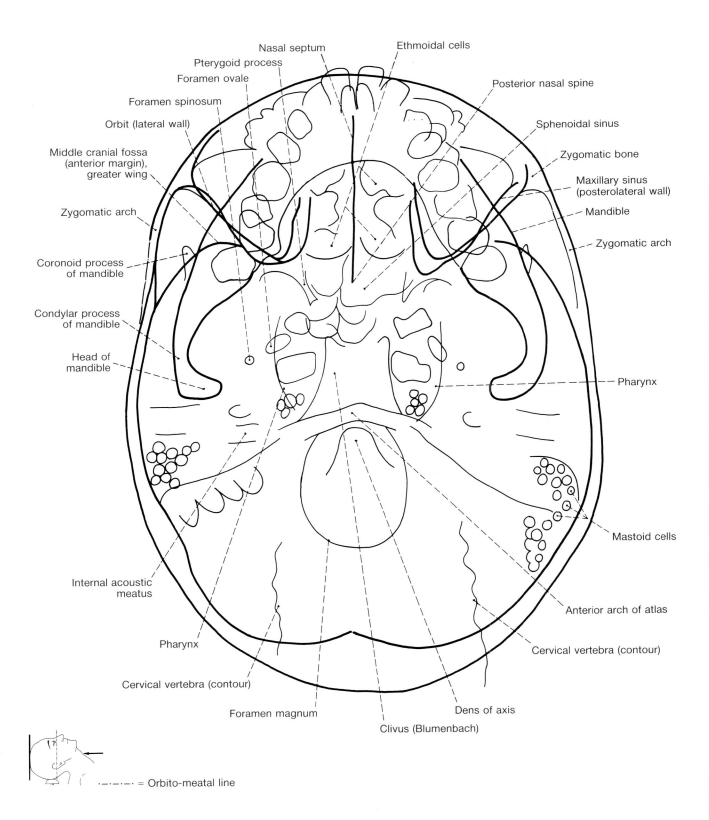

Nasal septum

Ethmoidal cells

Pterygoid process

Foramen ovale

Posterior nasal spine

Foramen spinosum

Sphenoidal sinus

Orbit (lateral wall)

Zygomatic bone

Middle cranial fossa
(anterior margin),
greater wing

Maxillary sinus
(posterolateral wall)

Mandible

Zygomatic arch

Zygomatic arch

Coronoid process
of mandible

Condylar process
of mandible

Head of
mandible

Pharynx

Internal acoustic
meatus

Mastoid cells

Anterior arch of atlas

Pharynx

Cervical vertebra (contour)

Cervical vertebra (contour)

Dens of axis

Foramen magnum

Clivus (Blumenbach)

-·-·-·- = Orbito-meatal line

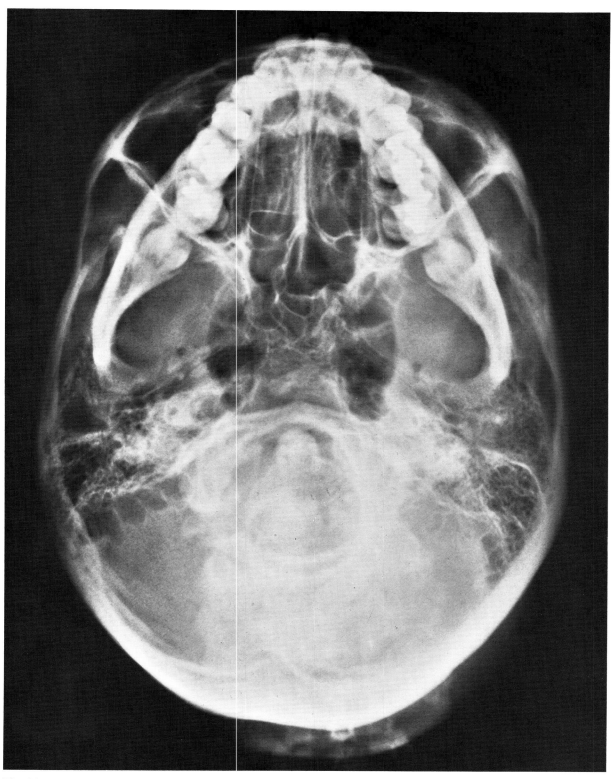

Fig. 14. Skull, axial view

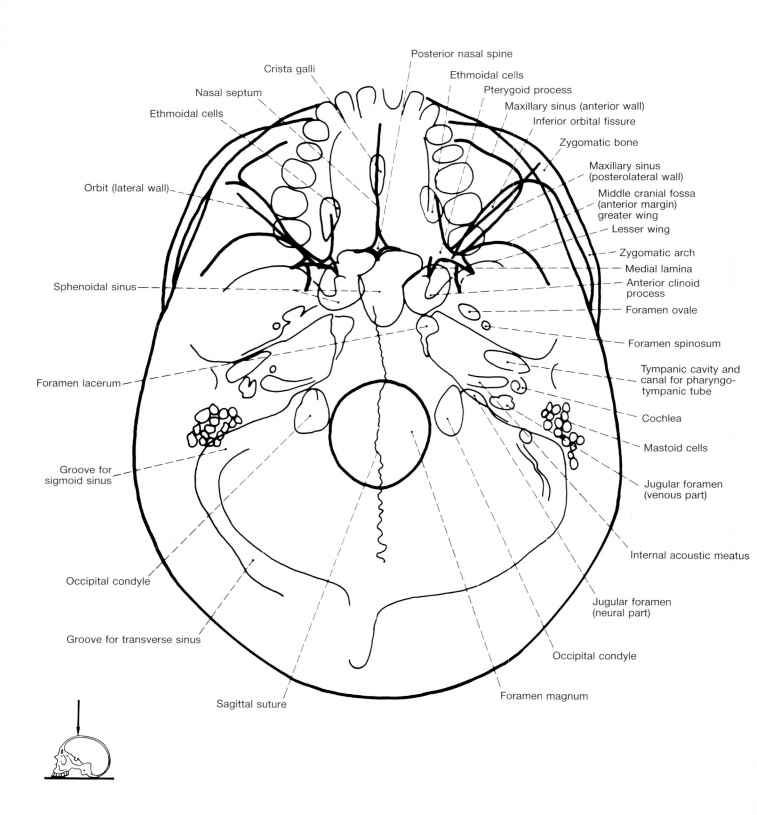

Posterior nasal spine

Crista galli

Ethmoidal cells

Nasal septum

Pterygoid process

Ethmoidal cells

Maxillary sinus (anterior wall)

Inferior orbital fissure

Zygomatic bone

Maxillary sinus (posterolateral wall)

Orbit (lateral wall)

Middle cranial fossa (anterior margin) greater wing

Lesser wing

Zygomatic arch

Medial lamina

Anterior clinoid process

Sphenoidal sinus

Foramen ovale

Foramen spinosum

Tympanic cavity and canal for pharyngo-tympanic tube

Foramen lacerum

Cochlea

Mastoid cells

Jugular foramen (venous part)

Groove for sigmoid sinus

Internal acoustic meatus

Occipital condyle

Jugular foramen (neural part)

Groove for transverse sinus

Occipital condyle

Sagittal suture

Foramen magnum

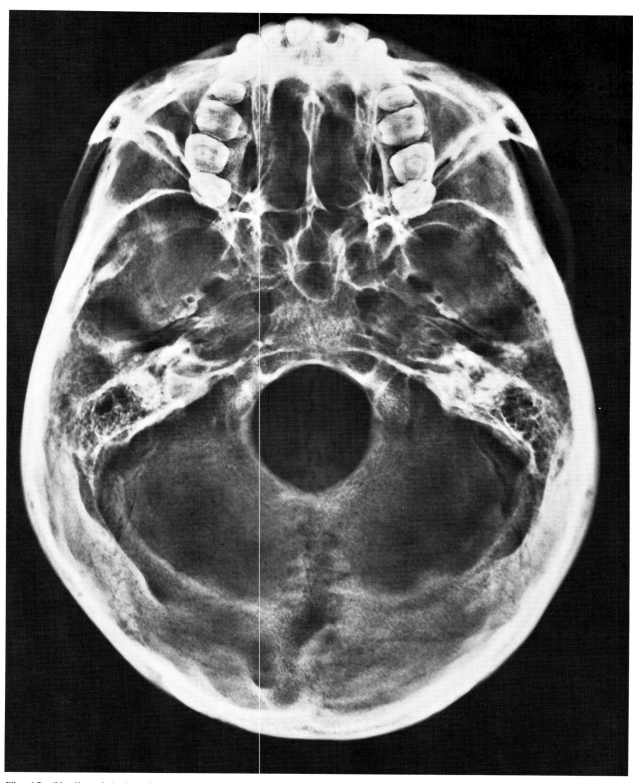

Fig. 15. Skull, axial view (skull from skeleton without mandible)

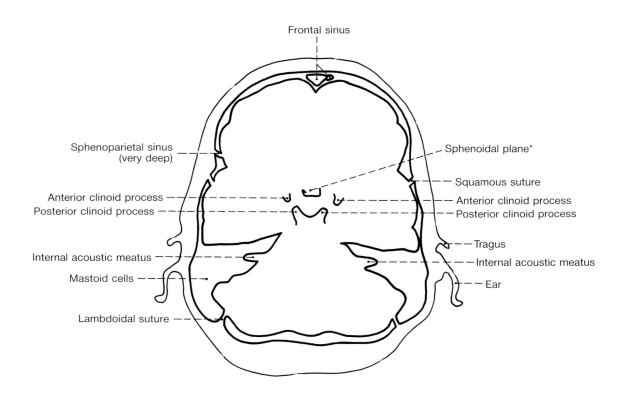

Frontal sinus

Sphenoparietal sinus
(very deep)

Sphenoidal plane*

Squamous suture

Anterior clinoid process

Anterior clinoid process

Posterior clinoid process

Posterior clinoid process

Tragus

Internal acoustic meatus

Internal acoustic meatus

Mastoid cells

Ear

Lambdoidal suture

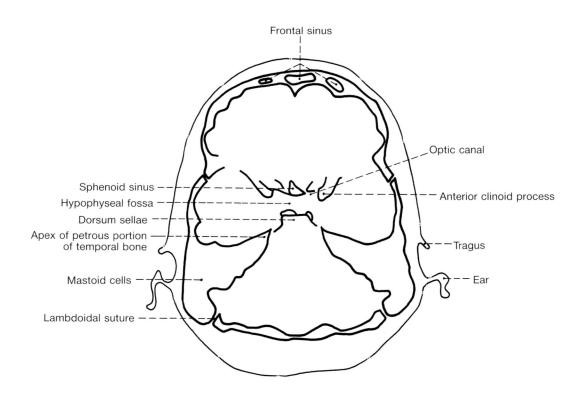

Frontal sinus

Optic canal

Sphenoid sinus

Anterior clinoid process

Hypophyseal fossa

Dorsum sellae

Apex of petrous portion
of temporal bone

Tragus

Mastoid cells

Ear

Lambdoidal suture

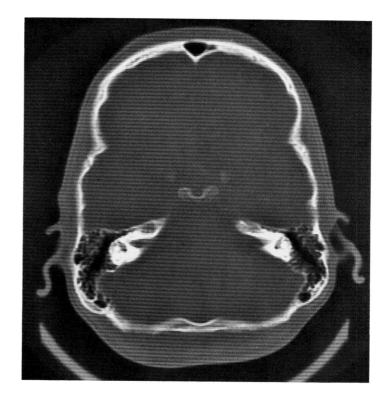

Fig. 16. Computed axial tomogram of skull

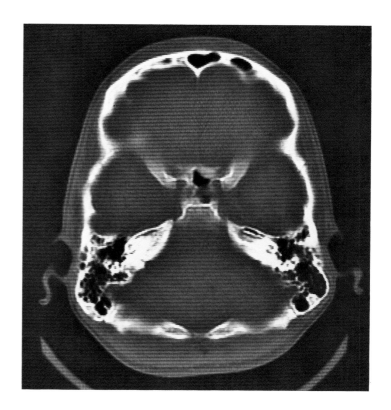

Fig. 17. Computed axial tomogram of skull

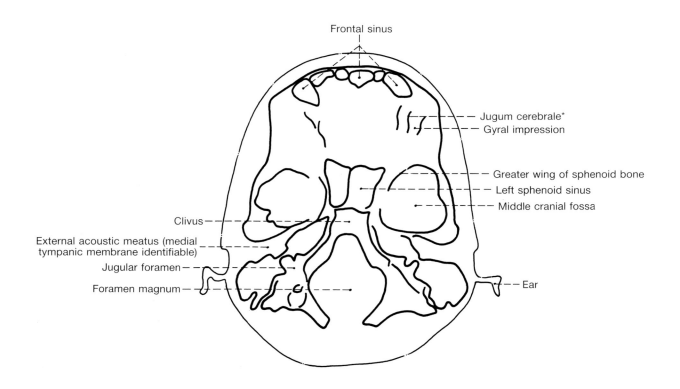

Frontal sinus

Jugum cerebrale*
Gyral impression

Greater wing of sphenoid bone
Left sphenoid sinus
Middle cranial fossa

Clivus

External acoustic meatus (medial tympanic membrane identifiable)

Jugular foramen

Foramen magnum

Ear

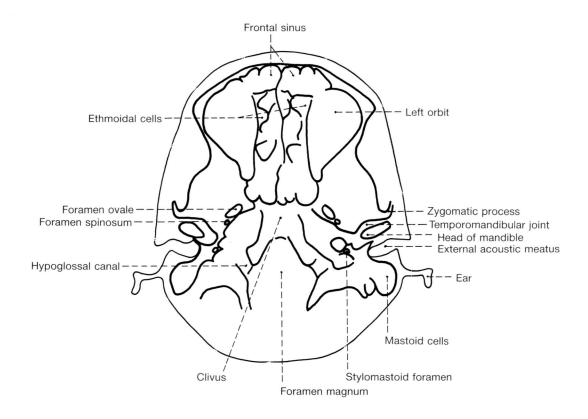

Frontal sinus

Ethmoidal cells

Left orbit

Foramen ovale
Foramen spinosum

Zygomatic process
Temporomandibular joint
Head of mandible
External acoustic meatus

Hypoglossal canal

Ear

Mastoid cells

Clivus

Stylomastoid foramen

Foramen magnum

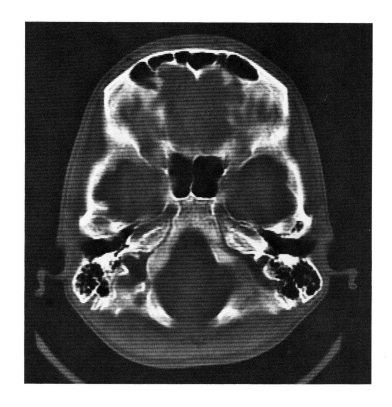

Fig. 18. Computed axial tomogram of skull

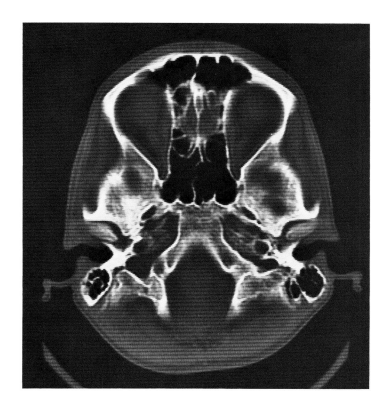

Fig. 19. Computed axial tomogram of skull

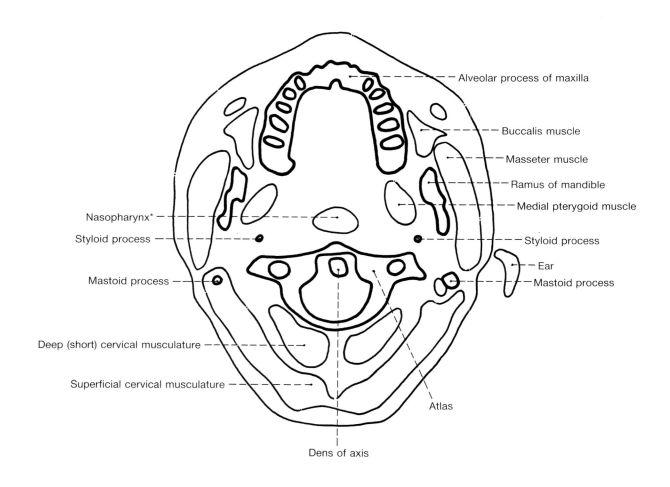

Alveolar process of maxilla

Buccalis muscle

Masseter muscle

Ramus of mandible

Medial pterygoid muscle

Nasopharynx*

Styloid process

Styloid process

Ear

Mastoid process

Mastoid process

Deep (short) cervical musculature

Superficial cervical musculature

Atlas

Dens of axis

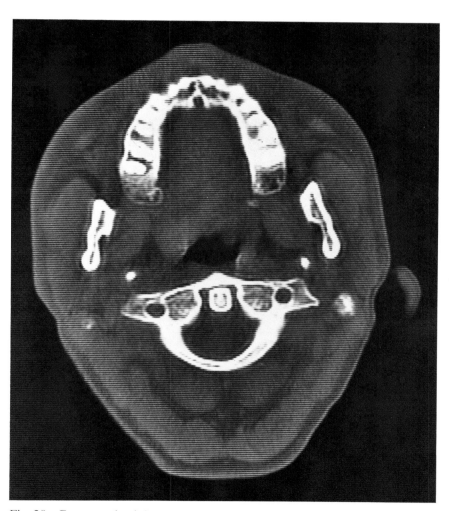

Fig. 20. Computed axial tomogram of skull

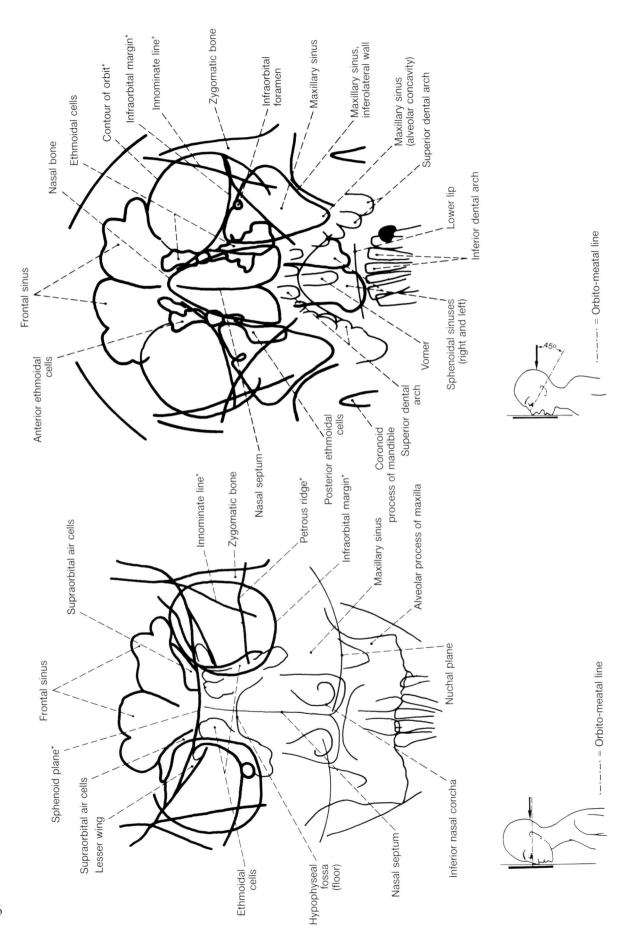

Contour of orbit*
Infraorbital margin*
Innominate line*
Zygomatic bone
Infraorbital foramen
Maxillary sinus
Maxillary sinus, inferolateral wall
Maxillary sinus (alveolar concavity)
Superior dental arch
Ethmoidal cells
Nasal bone
Lower lip
Inferior dental arch
Frontal sinus
Anterior ethmoidal cells
Vomer
Sphenoidal sinuses (right and left)
Superior dental arch
Coronoid process of mandible
Posterior ethmoidal cells
Infraorbital margin*
Nasal septum
Petrous ridge*
Zygomatic bone
Innominate line*
Supraorbital air cells
Maxillary sinus
Alveolar process of maxilla
Nuchal plane
Frontal sinus
Sphenoid plane*
Supraorbital air cells
Lesser wing
Ethmoidal cells
Hypophyseal fossa (floor)
Nasal septum
Inferior nasal concha

= Orbito-meatal line

= Orbito-meatal line

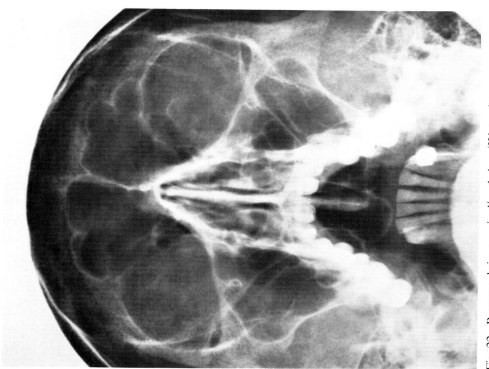

Fig. 22. Paranasal sinuses, inclined view (Waters)

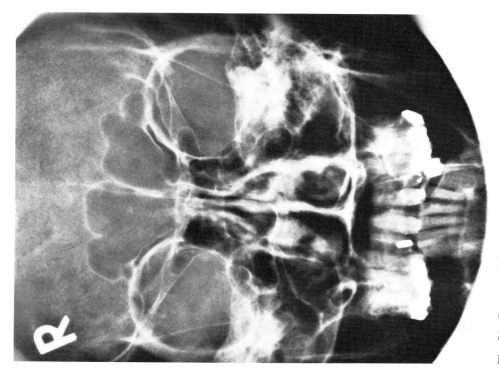

Fig. 21. Paranasal sinuses, p.a. view

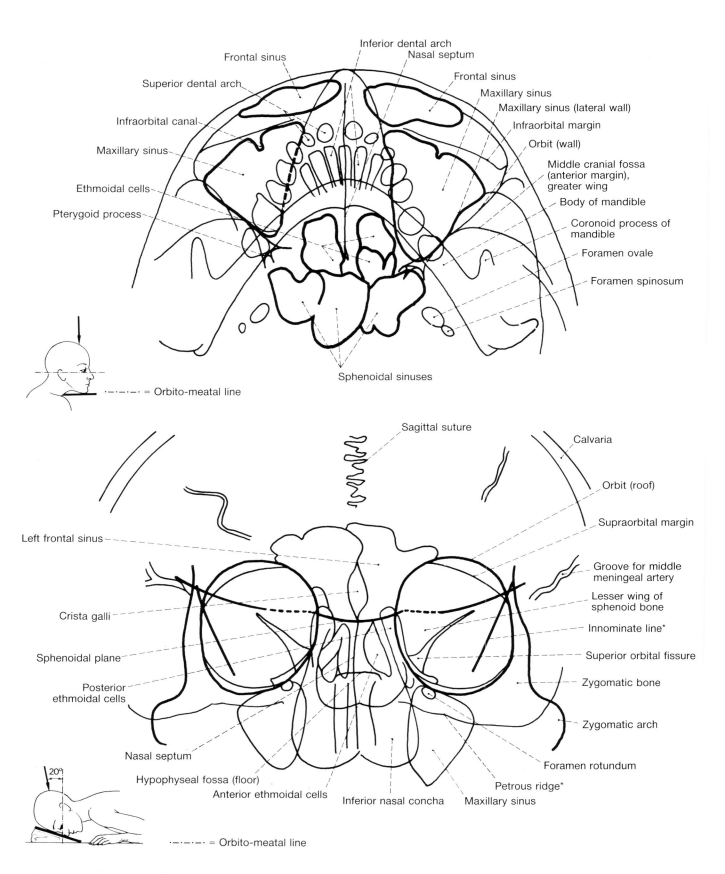

Inferior dental arch
Nasal septum
Frontal sinus
Superior dental arch
Frontal sinus
Maxillary sinus
Maxillary sinus (lateral wall)
Infraorbital canal
Infraorbital margin
Maxillary sinus
Orbit (wall)
Ethmoidal cells
Middle cranial fossa (anterior margin), greater wing
Pterygoid process
Body of mandible
Coronoid process of mandible
Foramen ovale
Foramen spinosum
Sphenoidal sinuses

—·—·— = Orbito-meatal line

Sagittal suture
Calvaria
Orbit (roof)
Supraorbital margin
Left frontal sinus
Groove for middle meningeal artery
Lesser wing of sphenoid bone
Crista galli
Innominate line*
Sphenoidal plane
Superior orbital fissure
Posterior ethmoidal cells
Zygomatic bone
Zygomatic arch
Nasal septum
Foramen rotundum
Hypophyseal fossa (floor)
Petrous ridge*
Anterior ethmoidal cells
Inferior nasal concha
Maxillary sinus

20°

—·—·— = Orbito-meatal line

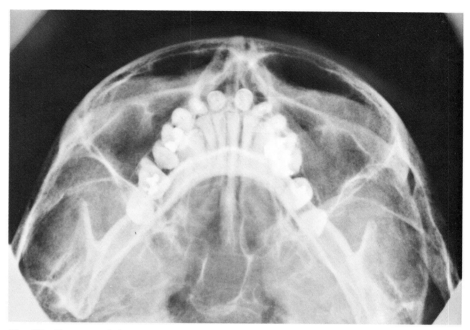

Fig. 23. Paranasal sinuses, half axial view

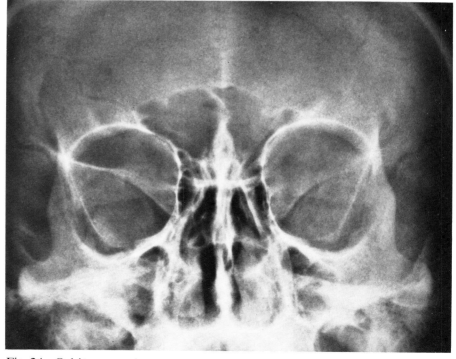

Fig. 24. Orbits, p.a. view

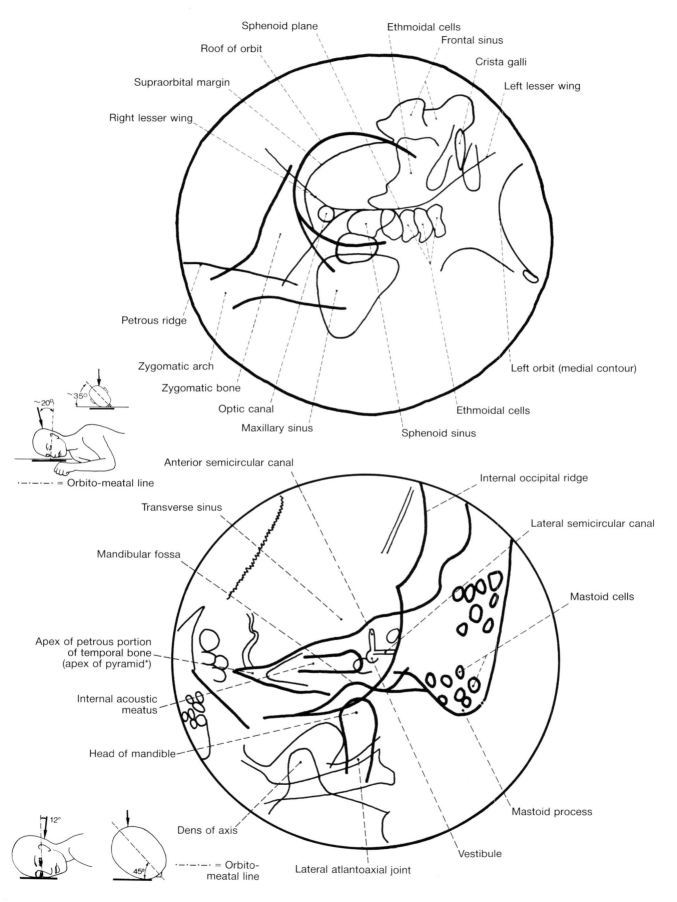

Sphenoid plane

Roof of orbit

Supraorbital margin

Right lesser wing

Ethmoidal cells

Frontal sinus

Crista galli

Left lesser wing

~20°

~35°

—·—·—· = Orbito-meatal line

Petrous ridge

Zygomatic arch

Zygomatic bone

Optic canal

Maxillary sinus

Sphenoid sinus

Ethmoidal cells

Left orbit (medial contour)

Anterior semicircular canal

Internal occipital ridge

Transverse sinus

Lateral semicircular canal

Mandibular fossa

Mastoid cells

Apex of petrous portion
of temporal bone
(apex of pyramid*)

Internal acoustic
meatus

Head of mandible

12°

45°

—·—·—· = Orbito-
meatal line

Dens of axis

Lateral atlantoaxial joint

Vestibule

Mastoid process

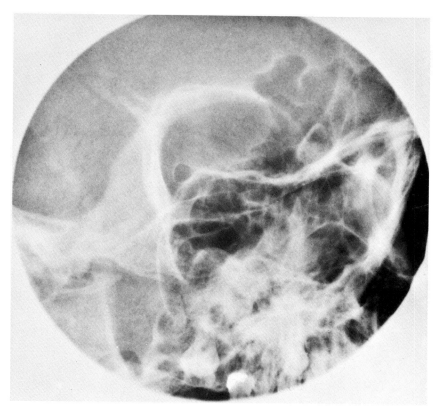

Fig. 25. Radiograph of right
optic canal (Rhese)

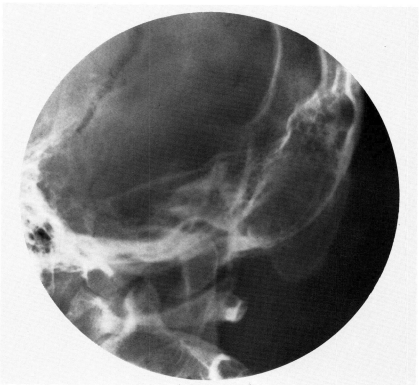

Fig. 26. Semisagittal radiograph
of right temporal bone (Stenvers)

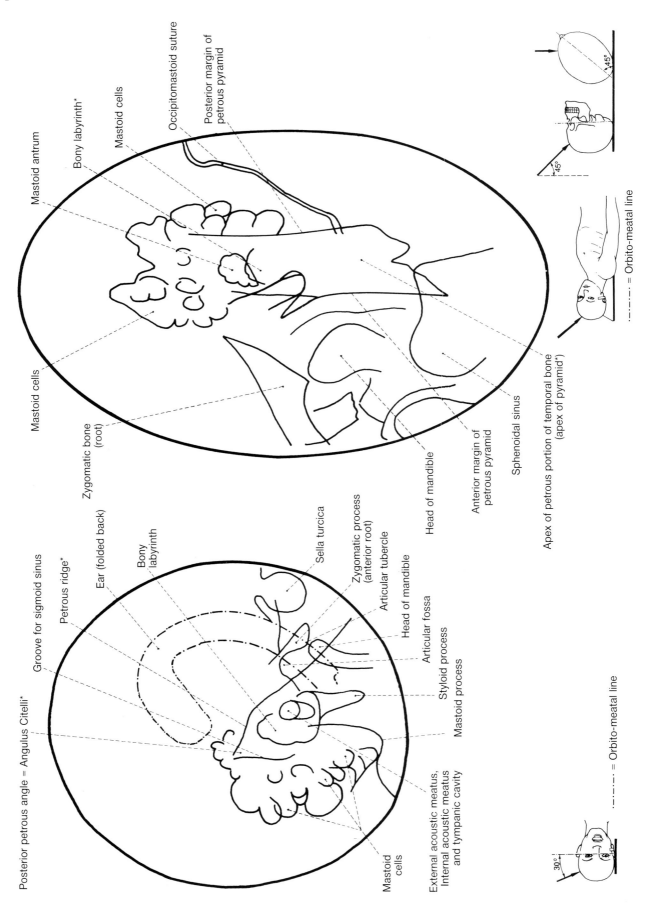

Mastoid antrum

Bony labyrinth*

Mastoid cells

Occipitomastoid suture

Posterior margin of petrous pyramid

Mastoid cells

Zygomatic bone (root)

Ear (folded back)

Bony labyrinth

Sella turcica

Zygomatic process (anterior root)

Articular tubercle

Head of mandible

Articular fossa

Styloid process

Mastoid process

Head of mandible

Anterior margin of petrous pyramid

Sphenoidal sinus

Apex of petrous portion of temporal bone (apex of pyramid*)

Posterior petrous angle = Angulus Citelli*

Groove for sigmoid sinus

Petrous ridge*

Mastoid cells

External acoustic meatus, Internal acoustic meatus and tympanic cavity

-·-·- = Orbito-meatal line

-·-·- = Orbito-meatal line

45°

45°

30°

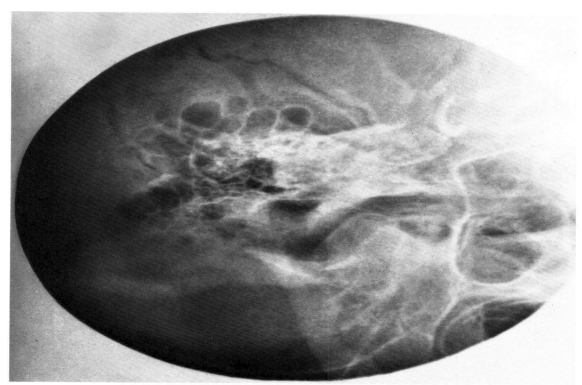

Fig. 28. Radiograph of left temporal bone, half axial view (Mayer)

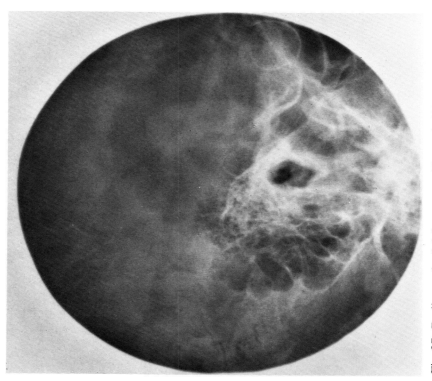

Fig. 27. Radiograph of right temporal bone, half lateral view (Schüller)

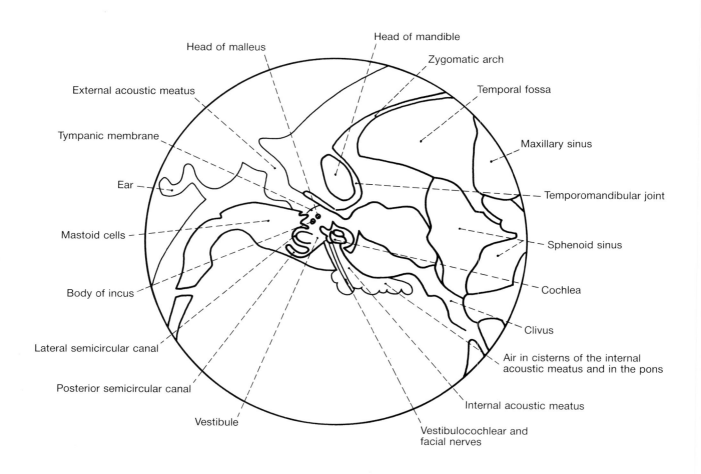

Head of malleus

Head of mandible

Zygomatic arch

External acoustic meatus

Temporal fossa

Tympanic membrane

Maxillary sinus

Ear

Temporomandibular joint

Mastoid cells

Sphenoid sinus

Body of incus

Cochlea

Lateral semicircular canal

Clivus

Posterior semicircular canal

Air in cisterns of the internal
acoustic meatus and in the pons

Vestibule

Internal acoustic meatus

Vestibulocochlear and
facial nerves

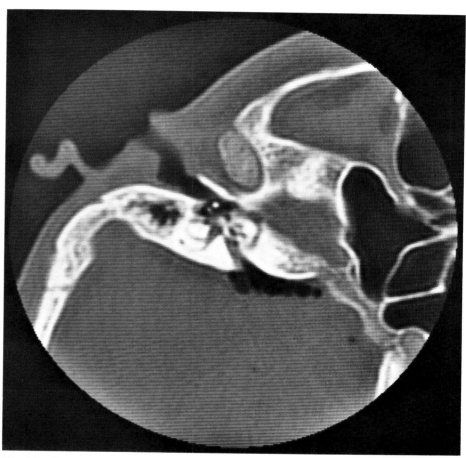

Fig. 29. Computed axial tomogram of right petrous bone (pneumocisternography)

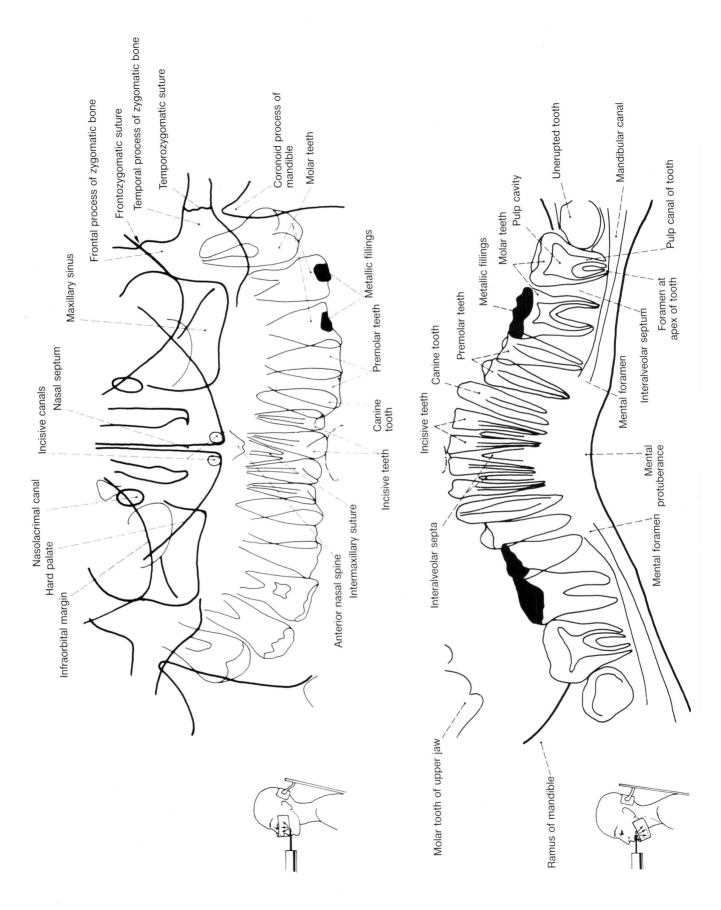

Frontal process of zygomatic bone
Frontozygomatic suture
Temporal process of zygomatic bone
Temporozygomatic suture
Coronoid process of mandible
Molar teeth
Maxillary sinus
Metallic fillings
Nasal septum
Incisive canals
Premolar teeth
Nasolacrimal canal
Canine tooth
Hard palate
Incisive teeth
Infraorbital margin
Anterior nasal spine
Intermaxillary suture

Unerupted tooth
Mandibular canal
Pulp cavity
Molar teeth
Metallic fillings
Pulp canal of tooth
Premolar teeth
Canine tooth
Foramen at apex of tooth
Incisive teeth
Interalveolar septum
Mental foramen
Interalveolar septa
Mental protuberance
Mental foramen

Molar tooth of upper jaw

Ramus of mandible

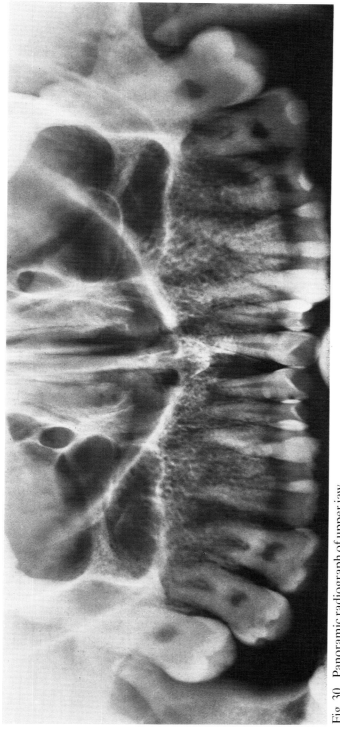

Fig. 30. Panoramic radiograph of upper jaw

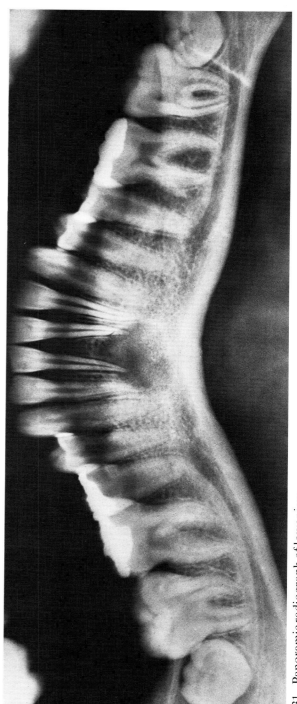

Fig. 31. Panoramic radiograph of lower jaw

Carotid Angiography

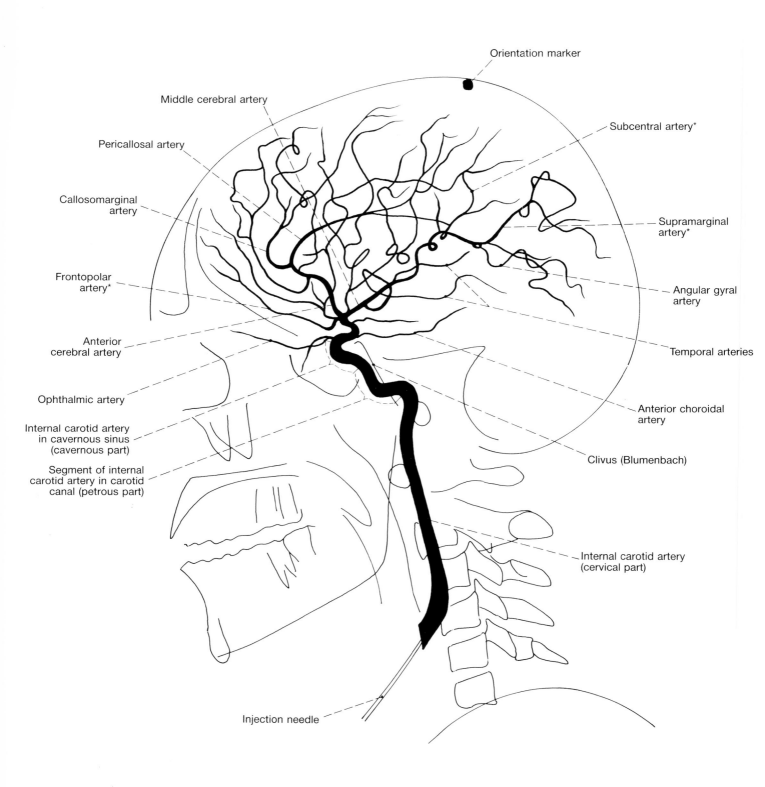

Orientation marker

Middle cerebral artery

Pericallosal artery

Subcentral artery*

Callosomarginal artery

Supramarginal artery*

Frontopolar artery*

Angular gyral artery

Anterior cerebral artery

Temporal arteries

Ophthalmic artery

Internal carotid artery in cavernous sinus (cavernous part)

Anterior choroidal artery

Segment of internal carotid artery in carotid canal (petrous part)

Clivus (Blumenbach)

Internal carotid artery (cervical part)

Injection needle

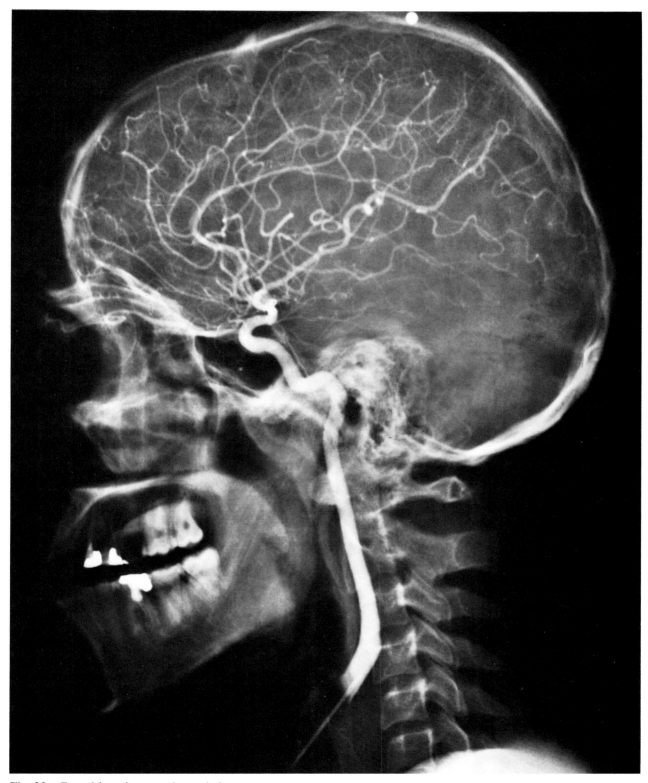

Fig. 32. Carotid angiogram, lateral view

Carotid Angiography

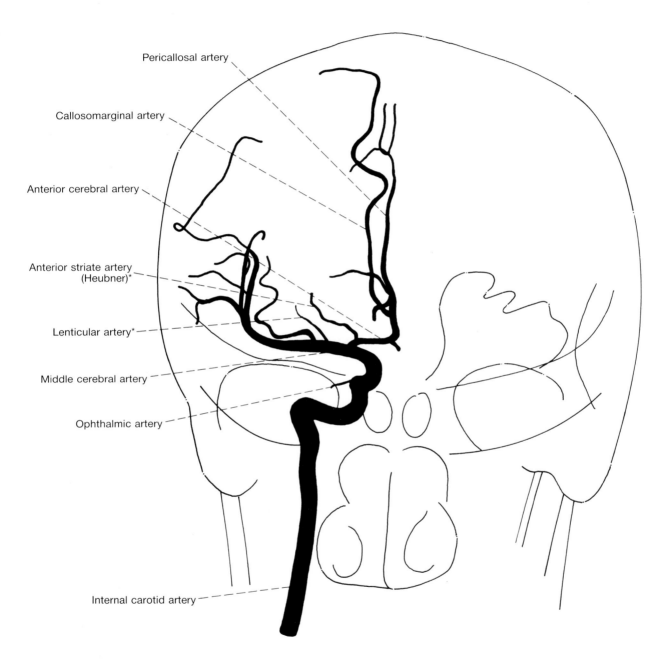

Pericallosal artery

Callosomarginal artery

Anterior cerebral artery

Anterior striate artery
(Heubner)*

Lenticular artery*

Middle cerebral artery

Ophthalmic artery

Internal carotid artery

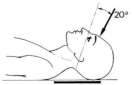

20°

–·–·–·– = Orbito-meatal line

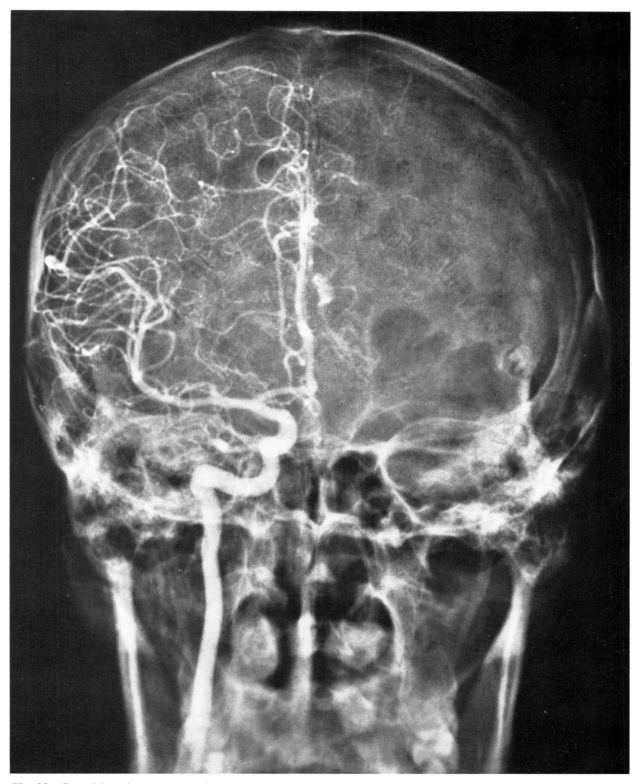

Fig. 33. Carotid angiogram, a.p. view

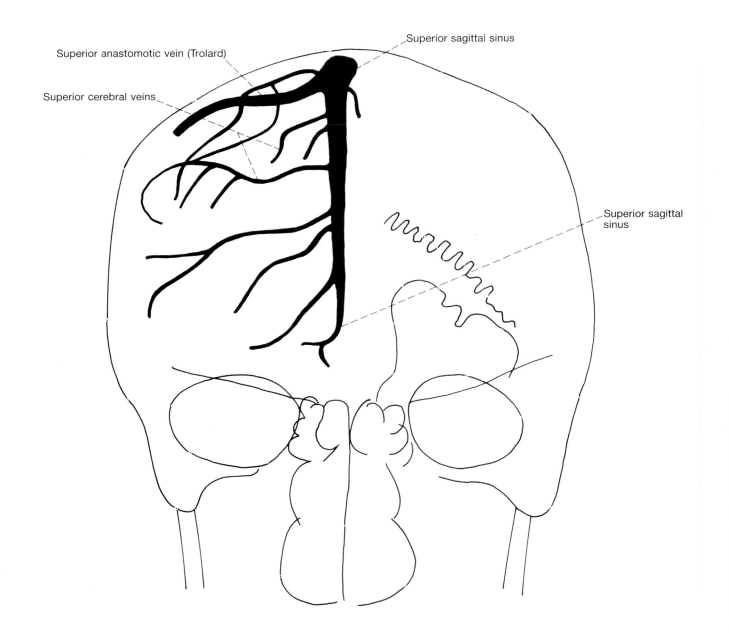

Superior sagittal sinus

Superior anastomotic vein (Trolard)

Superior cerebral veins

Superior sagittal sinus

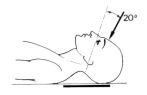

20°

—·—·—·— Orbito-meatal line

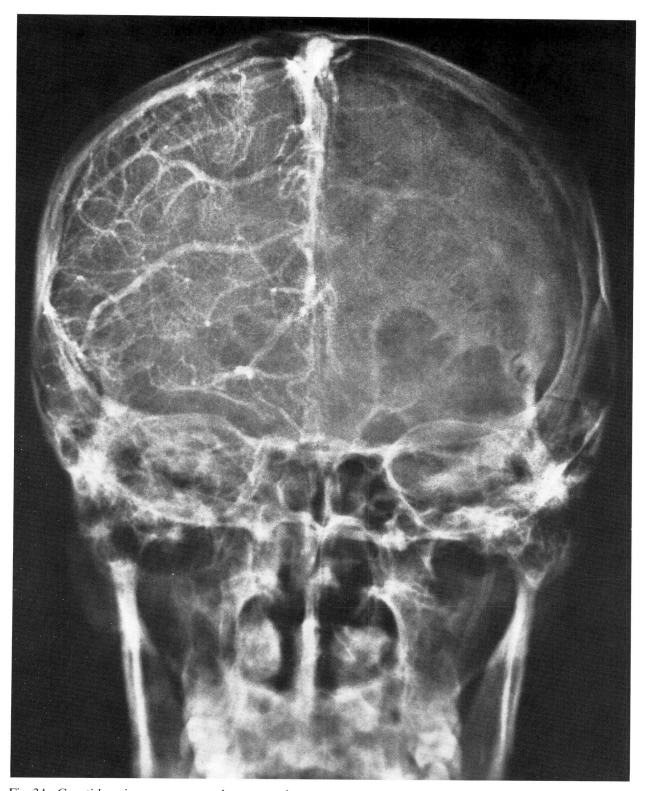

Fig. 34.   Carotid angiogram, venous phase, a.p. view

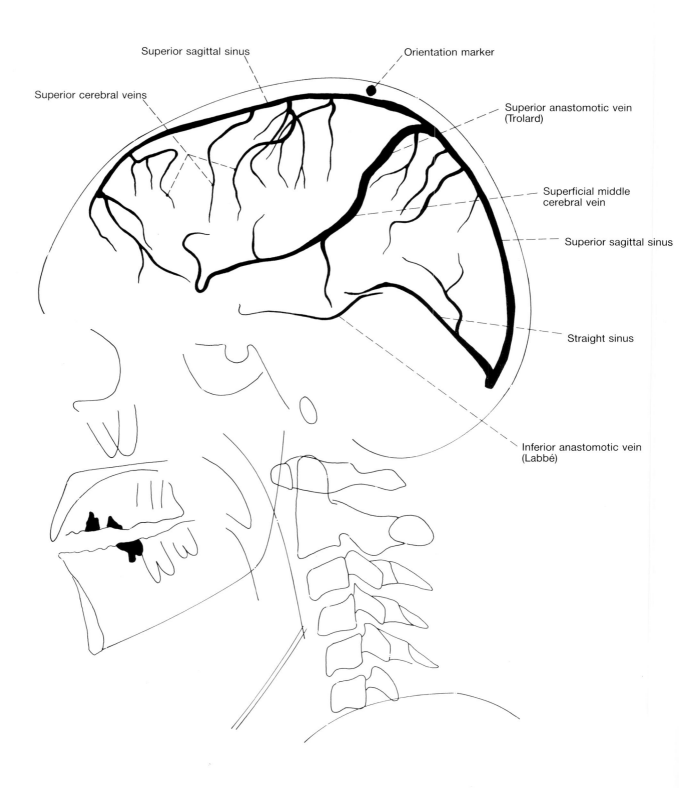

Superior sagittal sinus

Orientation marker

Superior cerebral veins

Superior anastomotic vein
(Trolard)

Superficial middle
cerebral vein

Superior sagittal sinus

Straight sinus

Inferior anastomotic vein
(Labbé)

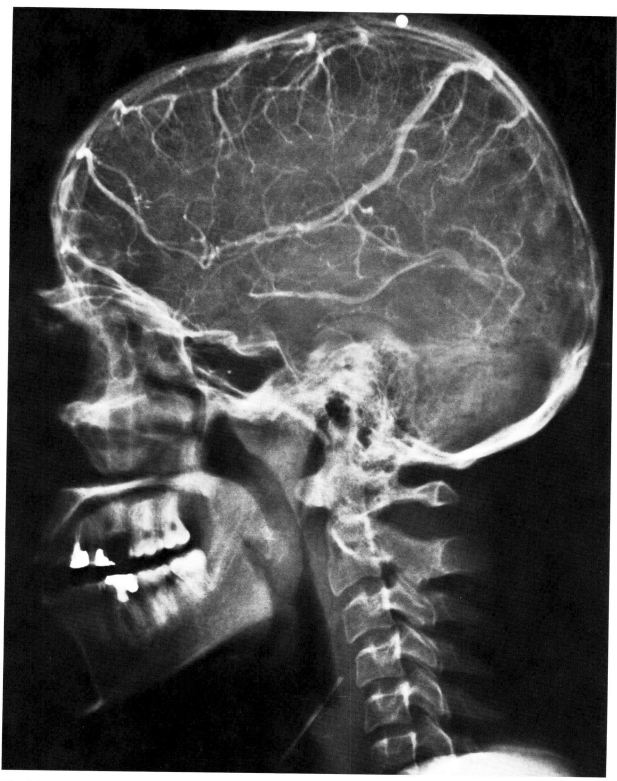

Fig. 35. Carotid angiogram, venous phase, lateral view

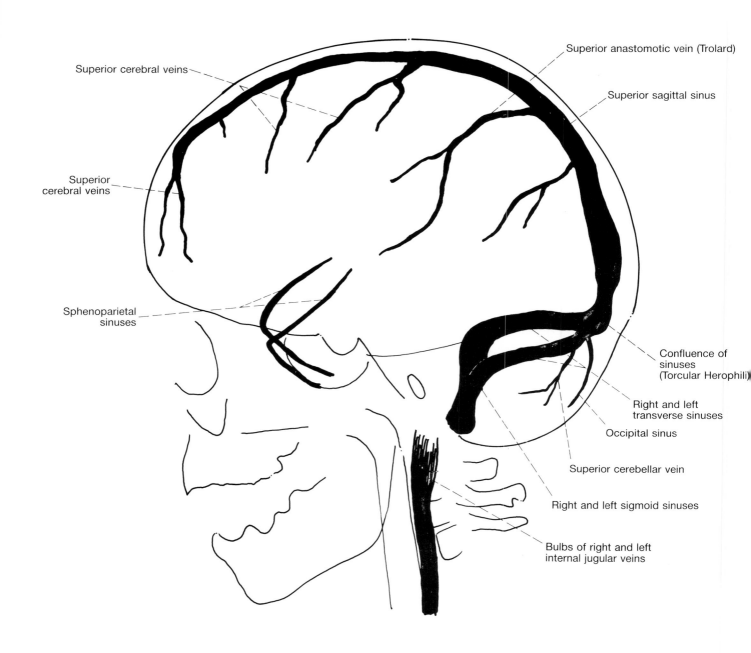

Superior cerebral veins

Superior cerebral veins

Sphenoparietal sinuses

Superior anastomotic vein (Trolard)

Superior sagittal sinus

Confluence of sinuses (Torcular Herophili)

Right and left transverse sinuses

Occipital sinus

Superior cerebellar vein

Right and left sigmoid sinuses

Bulbs of right and left internal jugular veins

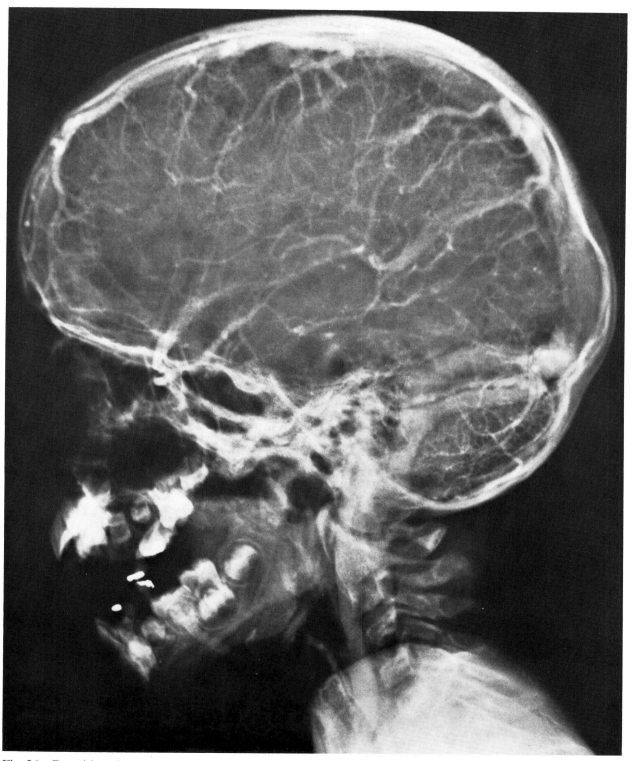

Fig. 36. Carotid angiogram, late venous phase, lateral view

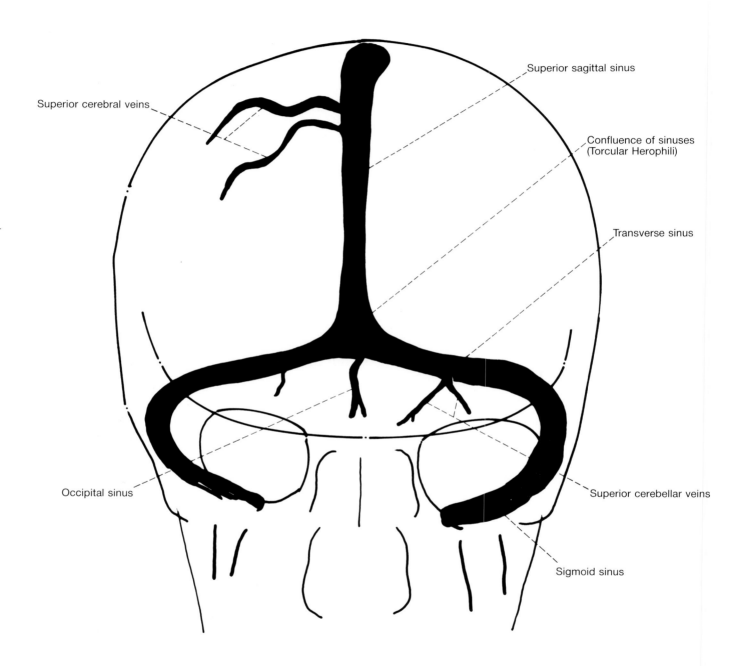

Superior sagittal sinus

Confluence of sinuses
(Torcular Herophili)

Transverse sinus

Superior cerebral veins

Superior cerebellar veins

Occipital sinus

Sigmoid sinus

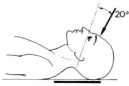

20°

·—·—·—· = Orbito-meatal line

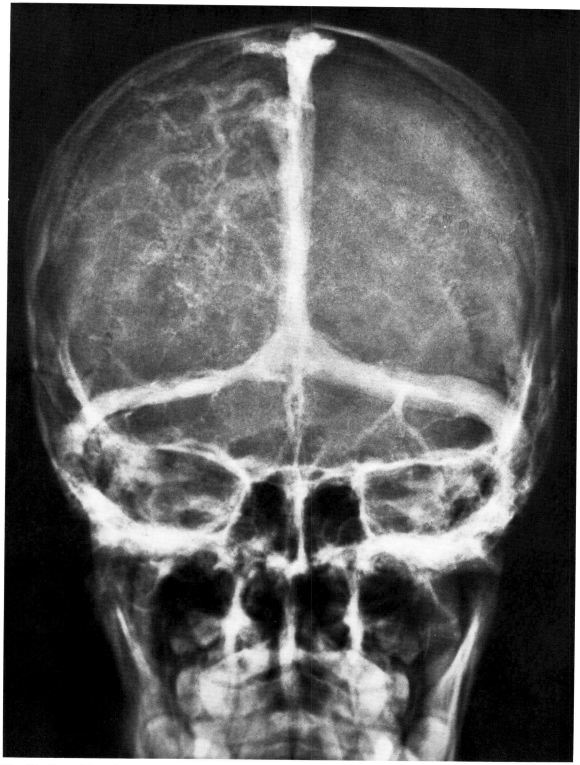

Fig. 37. Carotid angiogram, venous phase, a.p. view

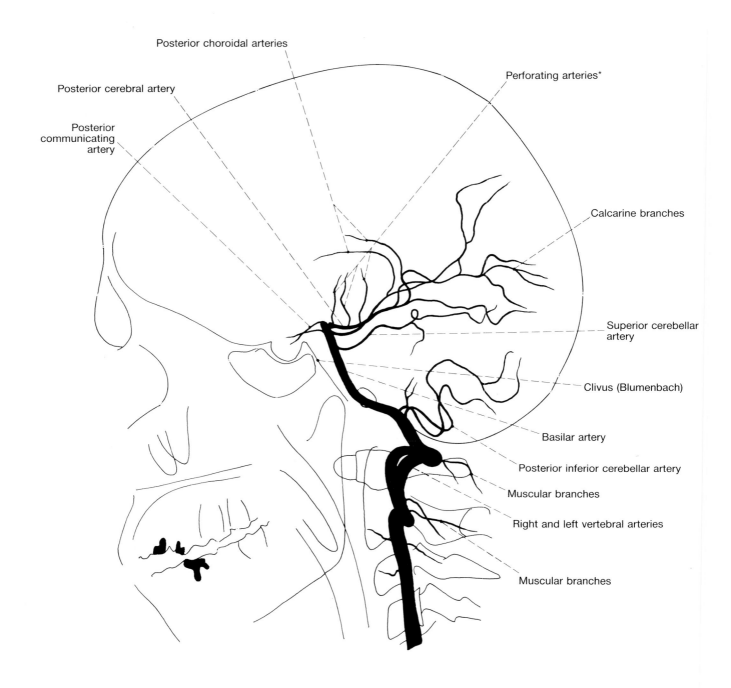

Posterior choroidal arteries

Perforating arteries*

Posterior cerebral artery

Posterior communicating artery

Calcarine branches

Superior cerebellar artery

Clivus (Blumenbach)

Basilar artery

Posterior inferior cerebellar artery

Muscular branches

Right and left vertebral arteries

Muscular branches

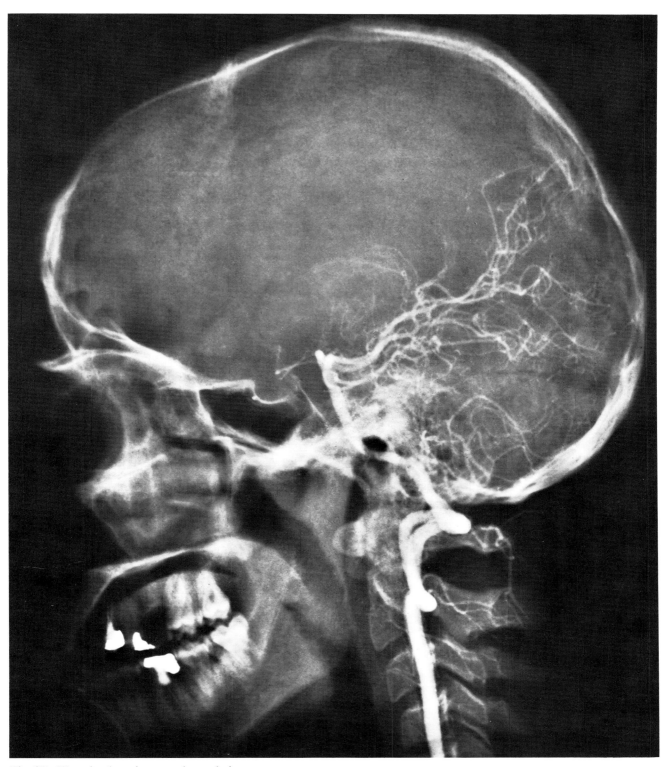

Fig. 38. Vertebral angiogram, lateral view

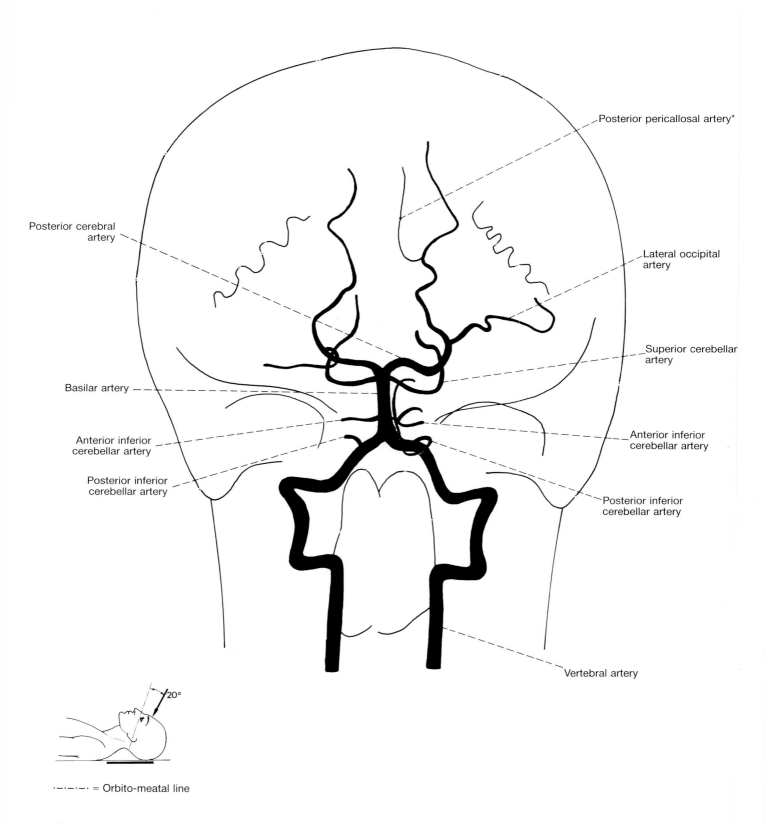

Posterior pericallosal artery*

Posterior cerebral artery

Lateral occipital artery

Superior cerebellar artery

Basilar artery

Anterior inferior cerebellar artery

Anterior inferior cerebellar artery

Posterior inferior cerebellar artery

Posterior inferior cerebellar artery

Vertebral artery

20°

—·—·—· = Orbito-meatal line

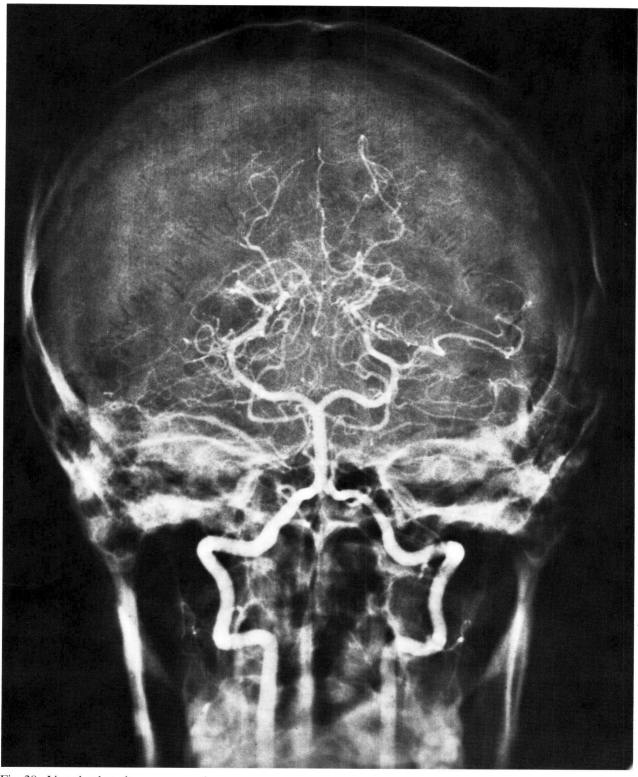

Fig. 39. Vertebral angiogram, a.p. view

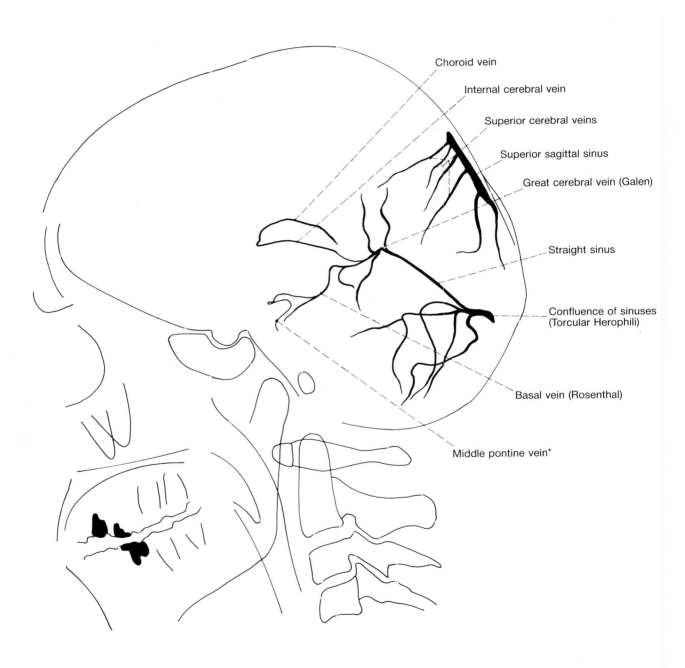

Choroid vein

Internal cerebral vein

Superior cerebral veins

Superior sagittal sinus

Great cerebral vein (Galen)

Straight sinus

Confluence of sinuses
(Torcular Herophili)

Basal vein (Rosenthal)

Middle pontine vein*

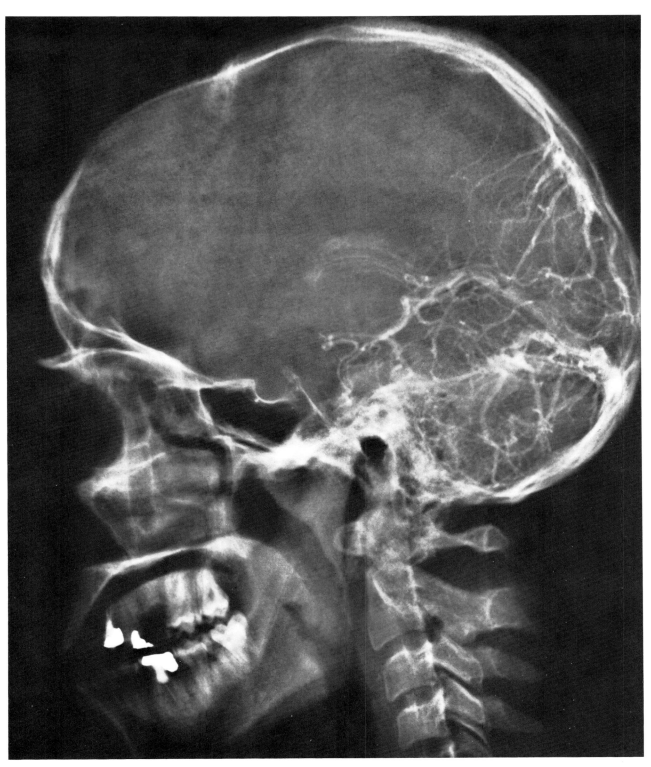

Fig. 40. Vertebral angiogram, venous phase, lateral view

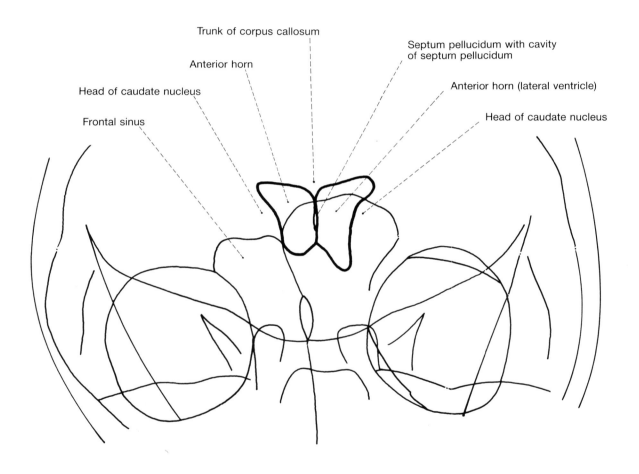

Trunk of corpus callosum

Anterior horn

Head of caudate nucleus

Frontal sinus

Septum pellucidum with cavity
of septum pellucidum

Anterior horn (lateral ventricle)

Head of caudate nucleus

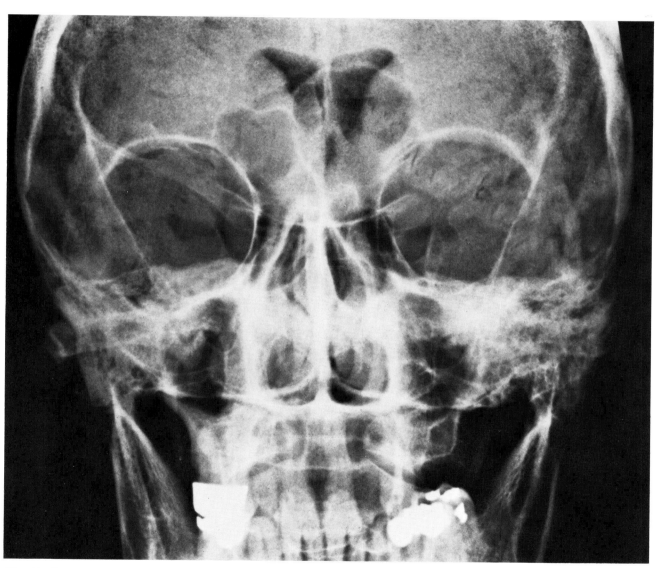

Fig. 41. Pneumoencephalogram, a.p. view

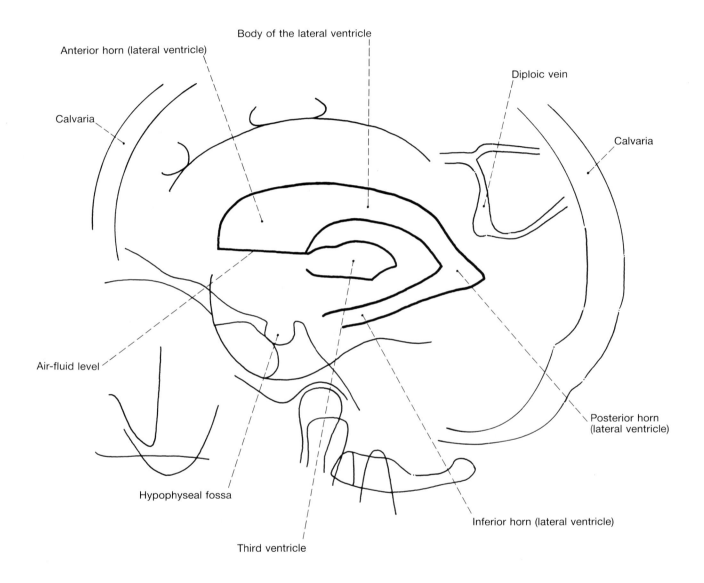

Anterior horn (lateral ventricle)

Body of the lateral ventricle

Diploic vein

Calvaria

Calvaria

Air-fluid level

Hypophyseal fossa

Third ventricle

Inferior horn (lateral ventricle)

Posterior horn (lateral ventricle)

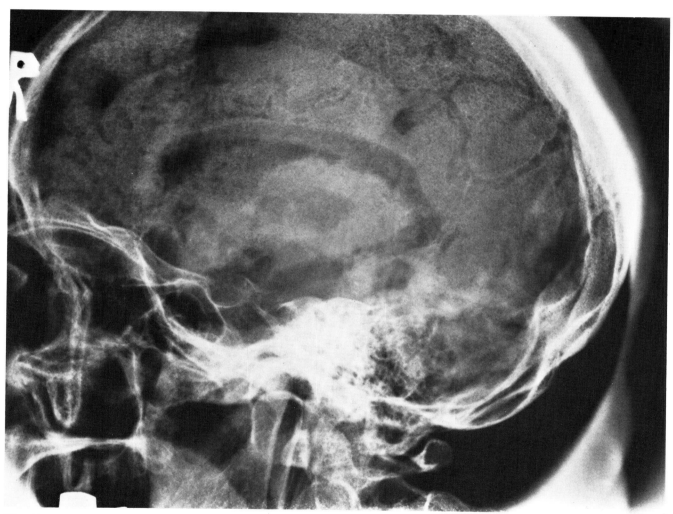

Fig. 42. Pneumoencephalogram, lateral view

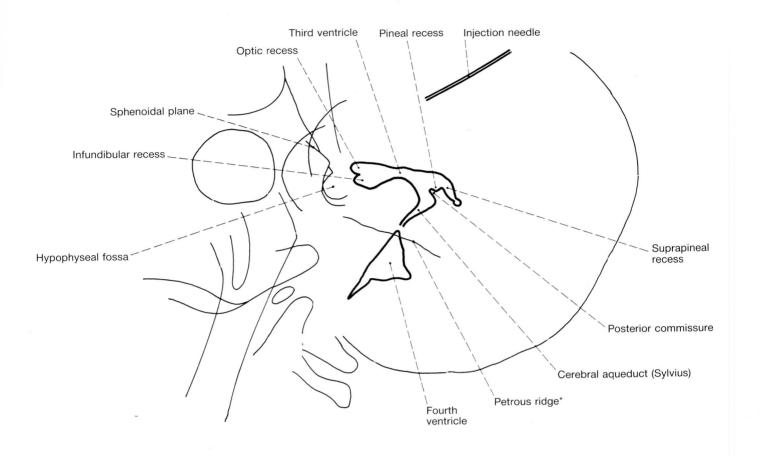

Optic recess — Third ventricle — Pineal recess — Injection needle

Sphenoidal plane

Infundibular recess

Hypophyseal fossa

Suprapineal recess

Posterior commissure

Cerebral aqueduct (Sylvius)

Fourth ventricle — Petrous ridge*

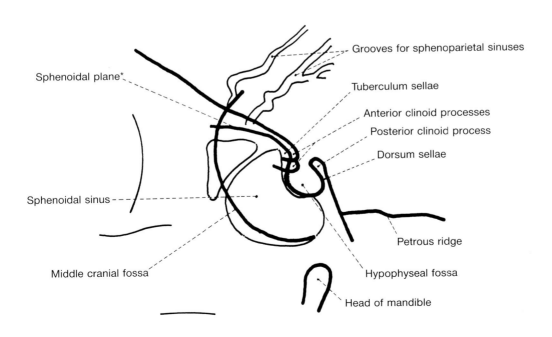

Grooves for sphenoparietal sinuses

Sphenoidal plane*

Tuberculum sellae

Anterior clinoid processes

Posterior clinoid process

Dorsum sellae

Sphenoidal sinus

Petrous ridge

Middle cranial fossa

Hypophyseal fossa

Head of mandible

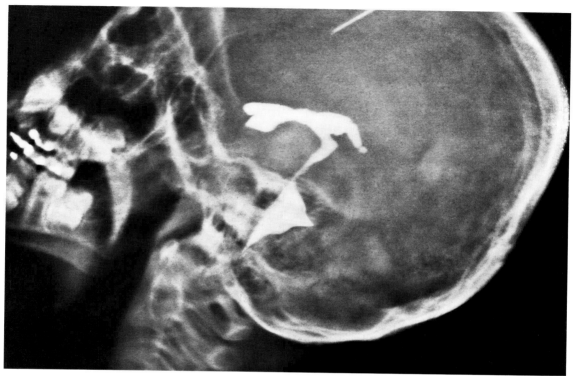

Fig. 43. Pantopaque ventriculogram

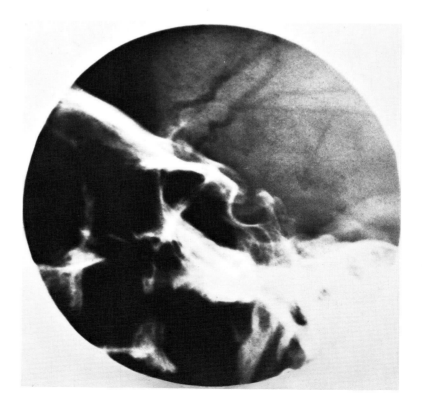

Fig. 44. Coned-down image of the sella turcica

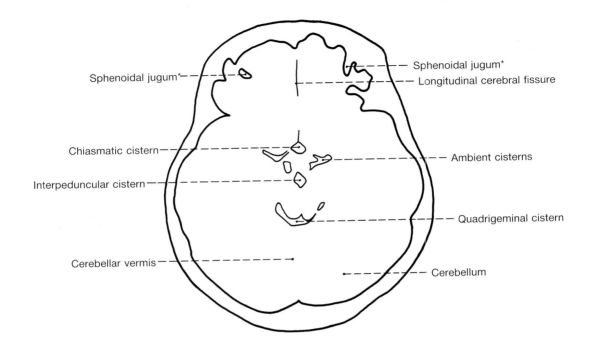

Sphenoidal jugum* — Sphenoidal jugum*

Longitudinal cerebral fissure

Chiasmatic cistern — Ambient cisterns

Interpeduncular cistern

Quadrigeminal cistern

Cerebellar vermis

Cerebellum

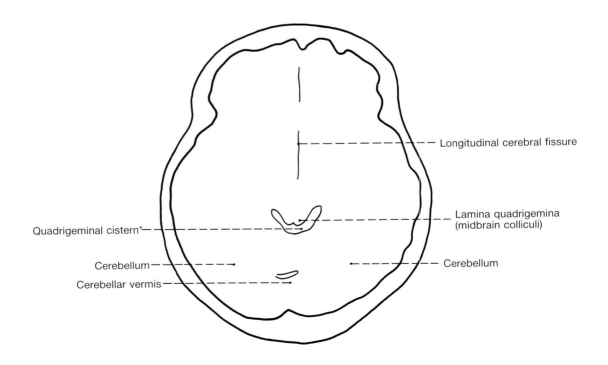

Longitudinal cerebral fissure

Lamina quadrigemina (midbrain colliculi)

Quadrigeminal cistern*

Cerebellum — Cerebellum

Cerebellar vermis

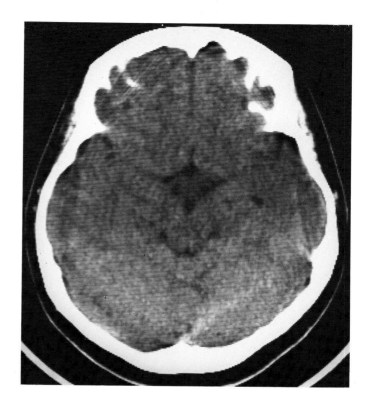

Fig. 45. Computed axial tomogram of the brain

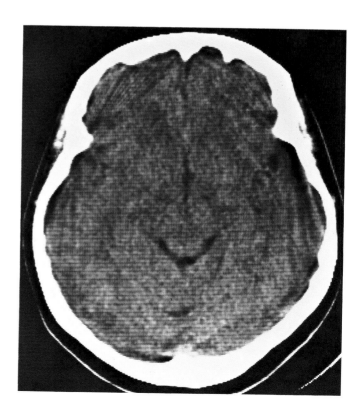

Fig. 46. Computed axial tomogram of the brain

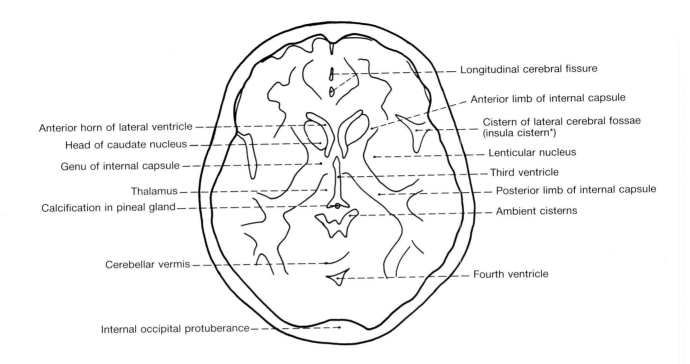

Longitudinal cerebral fissure

Anterior limb of internal capsule

Anterior horn of lateral ventricle

Head of caudate nucleus

Genu of internal capsule

Thalamus

Calcification in pineal gland

Cistern of lateral cerebral fossae (insula cistern*)

Lenticular nucleus

Third ventricle

Posterior limb of internal capsule

Ambient cisterns

Cerebellar vermis

Fourth ventricle

Internal occipital protuberance

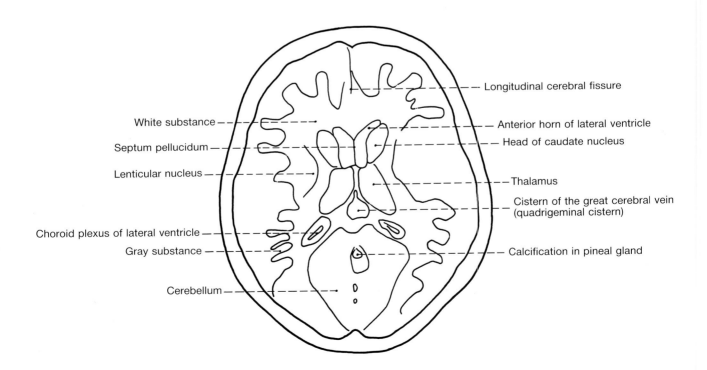

White substance

Septum pellucidum

Lenticular nucleus

Choroid plexus of lateral ventricle

Gray substance

Cerebellum

Longitudinal cerebral fissure

Anterior horn of lateral ventricle

Head of caudate nucleus

Thalamus

Cistern of the great cerebral vein (quadrigeminal cistern)

Calcification in pineal gland

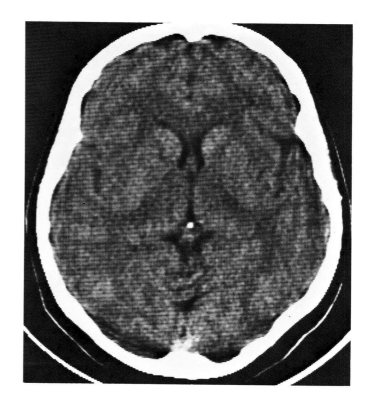

Fig. 47. Computed axial tomogram of the brain

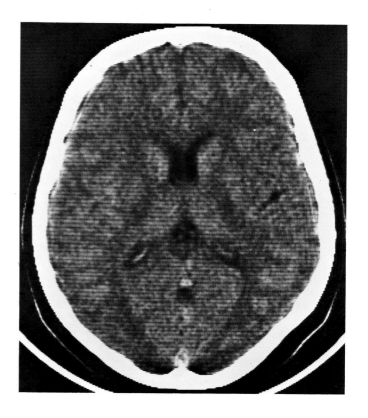

Fig. 48. Computed axial tomogram of the brain

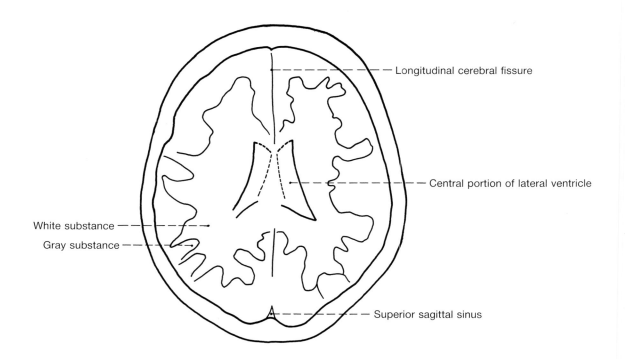

Longitudinal cerebral fissure

Central portion of lateral ventricle

White substance

Gray substance

Superior sagittal sinus

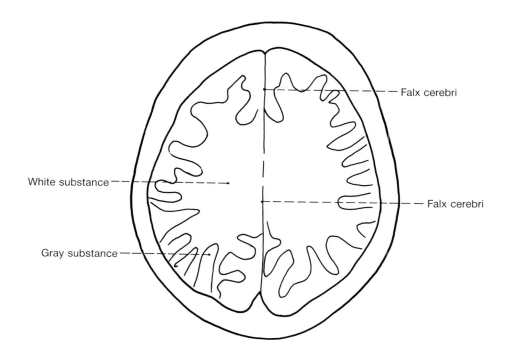

Falx cerebri

White substance

Falx cerebri

Gray substance

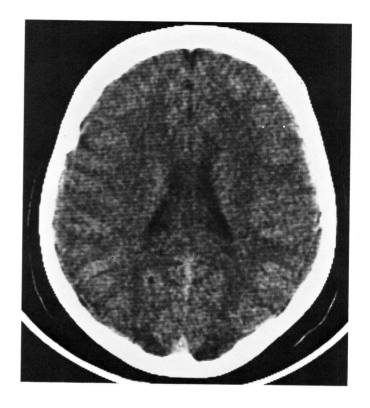

Fig. 49. Computed axial tomogram of the brain

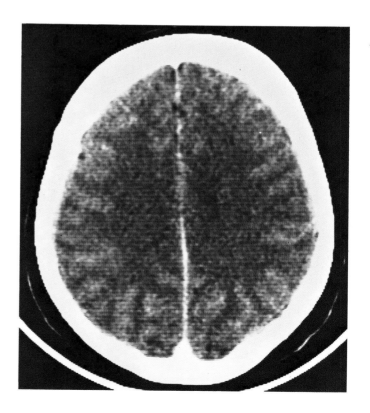

Fig. 50. Computed axial tomogram of the brain

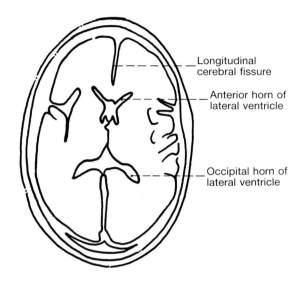

Longitudinal cerebral fissure

Anterior horn of lateral ventricle

Occipital horn of lateral ventricle

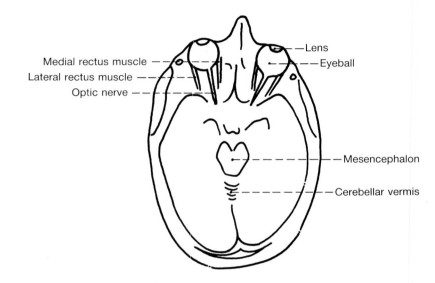

Lens

Medial rectus muscle

Lateral rectus muscle

Optic nerve

Eyeball

Mesencephalon

Cerebellar vermis

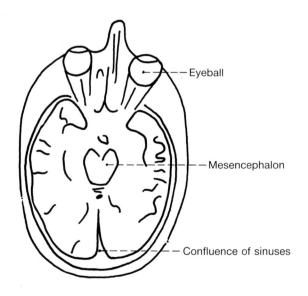

Eyeball

Mesencephalon

Confluence of sinuses

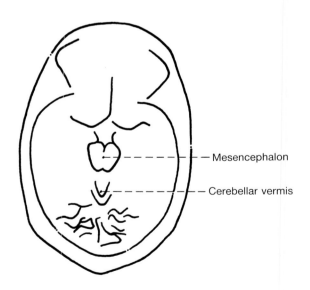

Mesencephalon

Cerebellar vermis

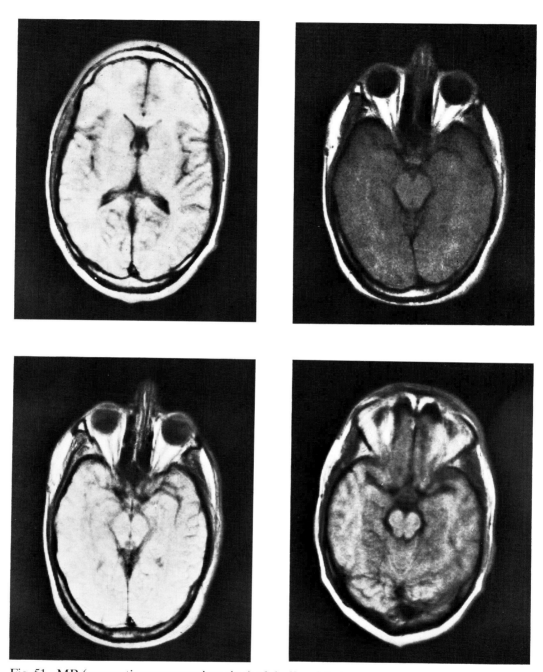

Fig. 51. MR (magnetic resonance imaging) of skull, axial views

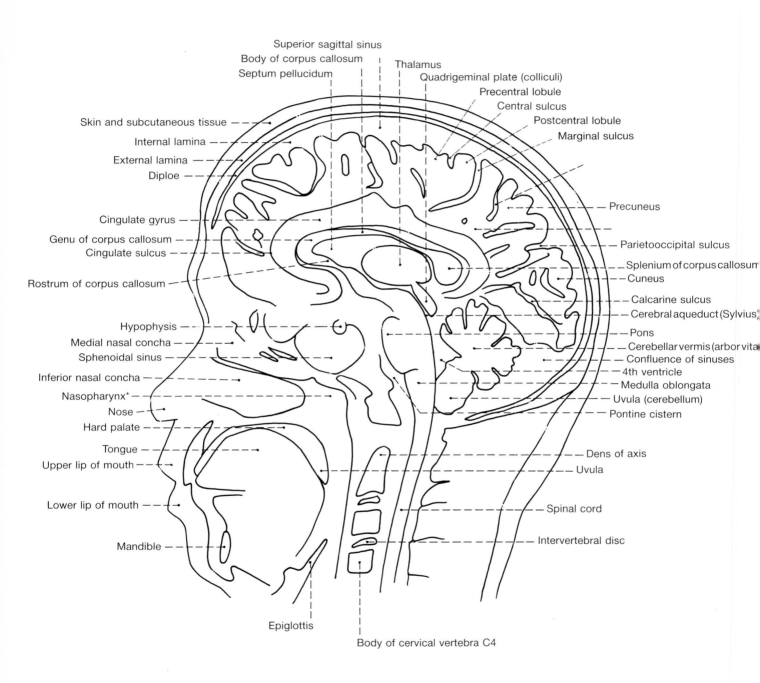

Superior sagittal sinus
Body of corpus callosum
Septum pellucidum
Thalamus
Quadrigeminal plate (colliculi)
Precentral lobule
Central sulcus
Postcentral lobule
Marginal sulcus

Skin and subcutaneous tissue
Internal lamina
External lamina
Diploe

Precuneus

Cingulate gyrus
Genu of corpus callosum
Cingulate sulcus

Parietooccipital sulcus
Splenium of corpus callosum
Cuneus

Rostrum of corpus callosum

Calcarine sulcus
Cerebral aqueduct (Sylvius)

Hypophysis
Medial nasal concha
Sphenoidal sinus

Pons
Cerebellar vermis (arbor vitae)
Confluence of sinuses
4th ventricle
Medulla oblongata
Uvula (cerebellum)
Pontine cistern

Inferior nasal concha
Nasopharynx*
Nose
Hard palate
Tongue
Upper lip of mouth

Dens of axis
Uvula

Lower lip of mouth

Spinal cord

Mandible

Intervertebral disc

Epiglottis

Body of cervical vertebra C4

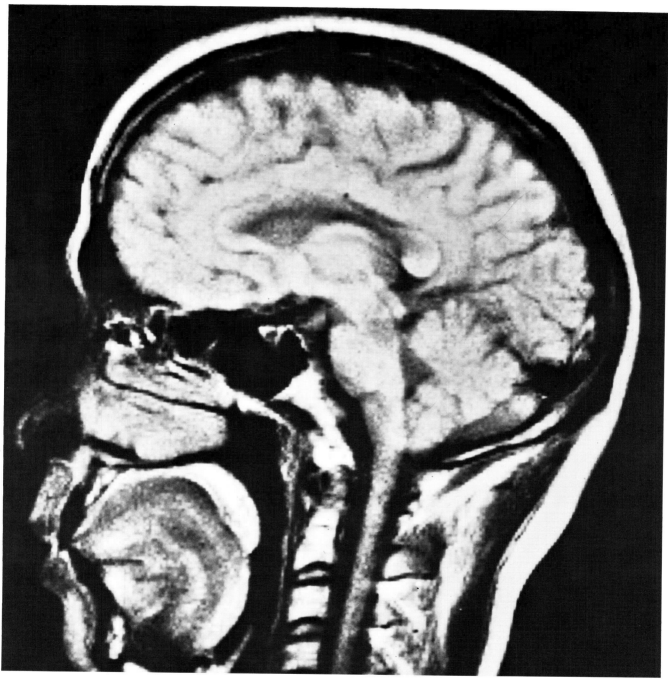

Fig. 52. Parasagittal section 5 mm from the sagittal plane, MR

Vertebral Column

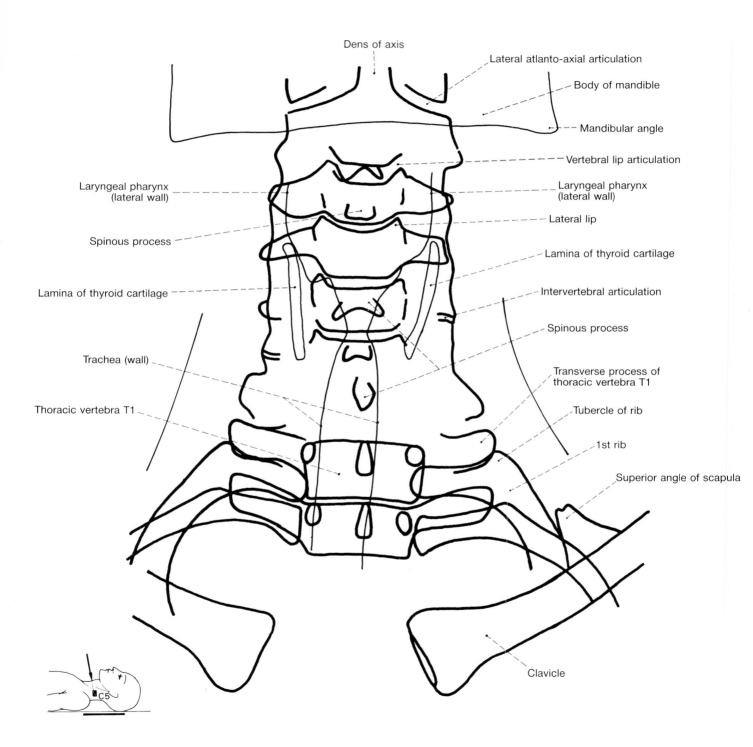

Dens of axis

Lateral atlanto-axial articulation

Body of mandible

Mandibular angle

Vertebral lip articulation

Laryngeal pharynx (lateral wall)

Laryngeal pharynx (lateral wall)

Lateral lip

Spinous process

Lamina of thyroid cartilage

Lamina of thyroid cartilage

Intervertebral articulation

Spinous process

Trachea (wall)

Transverse process of thoracic vertebra T1

Thoracic vertebra T1

Tubercle of rib

1st rib

Superior angle of scapula

Clavicle

C5

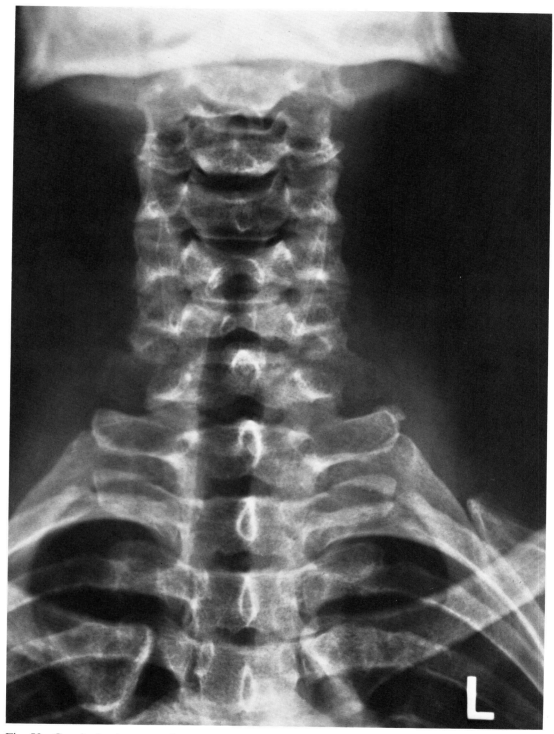

Fig. 53. Cervical spine, a.p. view

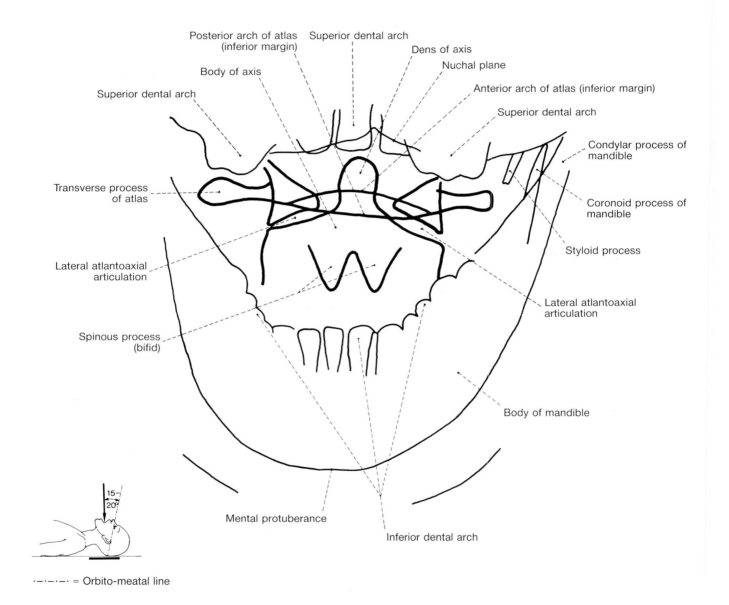

Posterior arch of atlas
(inferior margin)

Superior dental arch

Dens of axis

Nuchal plane

Body of axis

Anterior arch of atlas (inferior margin)

Superior dental arch

Superior dental arch

Condylar process of
mandible

Transverse process
of atlas

Coronoid process of
mandible

Styloid process

Lateral atlantoaxial
articulation

Lateral atlantoaxial
articulation

Spinous process
(bifid)

Body of mandible

Mental protuberance

Inferior dental arch

15
20°

·—·—·— · = Orbito-meatal line

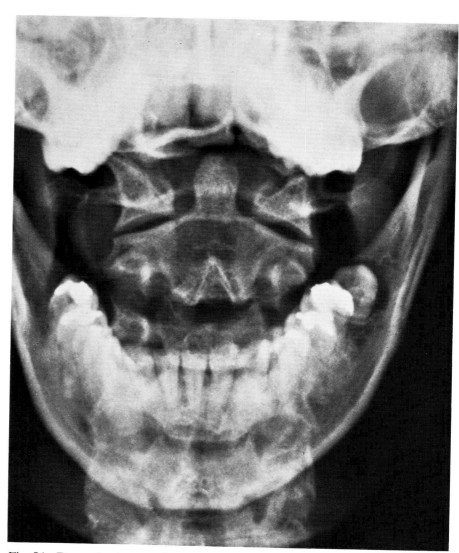

Fig. 54. Dens of axis, a.p. view

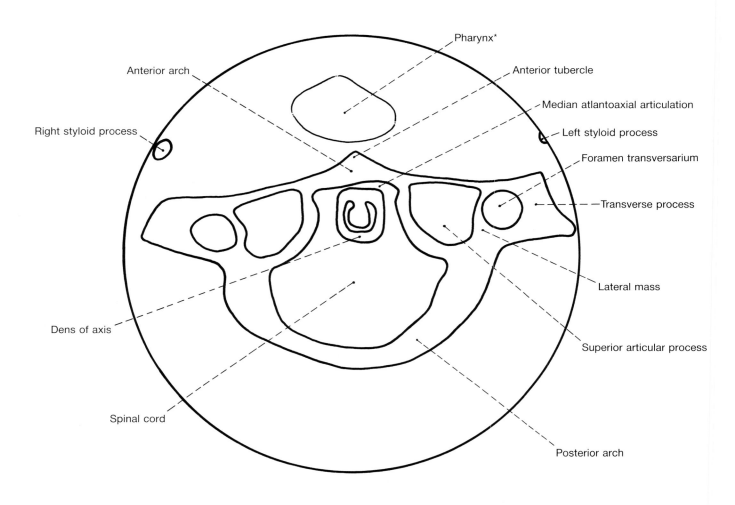

Pharynx*

Anterior arch

Anterior tubercle

Median atlantoaxial articulation

Right styloid process

Left styloid process

Foramen transversarium

Transverse process

Dens of axis

Lateral mass

Superior articular process

Spinal cord

Posterior arch

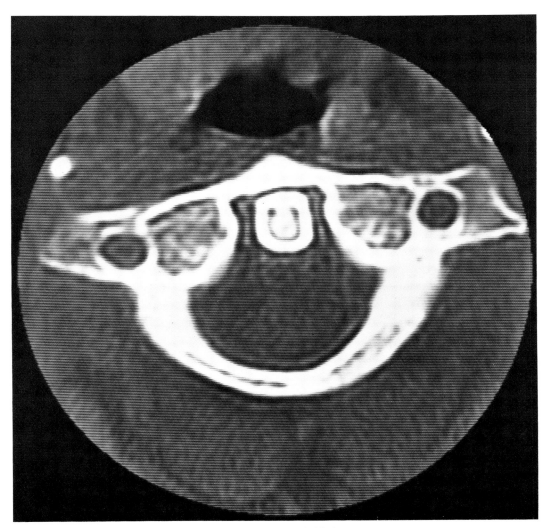

Fig. 55. Computed axial tomogram of the atlantoaxial joint

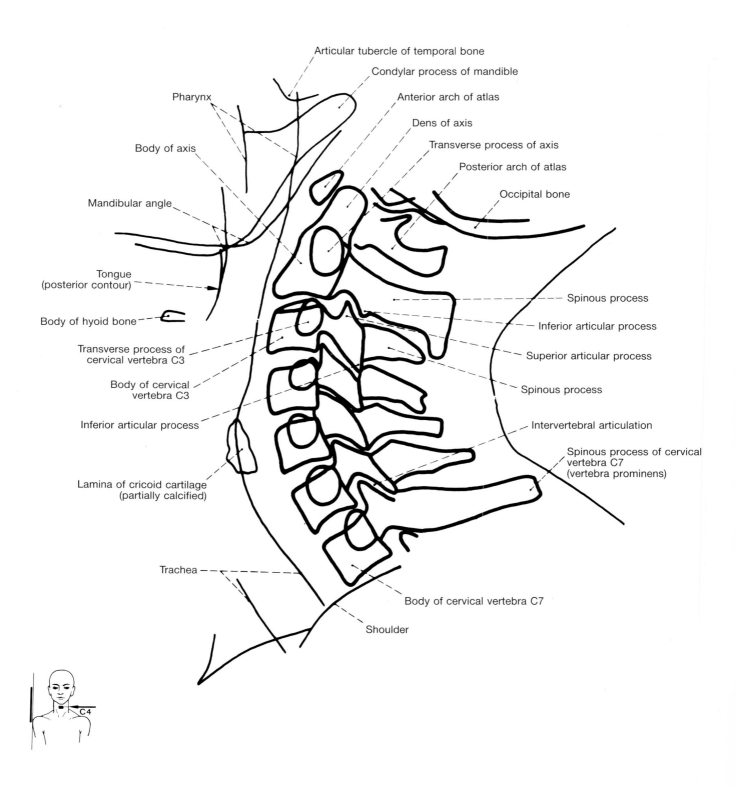

Articular tubercle of temporal bone

Condylar process of mandible

Anterior arch of atlas

Dens of axis

Transverse process of axis

Posterior arch of atlas

Occipital bone

Pharynx

Body of axis

Mandibular angle

Tongue
(posterior contour)

Body of hyoid bone

Transverse process of
cervical vertebra C3

Body of cervical
vertebra C3

Inferior articular process

Lamina of cricoid cartilage
(partially calcified)

Trachea

Spinous process

Inferior articular process

Superior articular process

Spinous process

Intervertebral articulation

Spinous process of cervical
vertebra C7
(vertebra prominens)

Body of cervical vertebra C7

Shoulder

C4

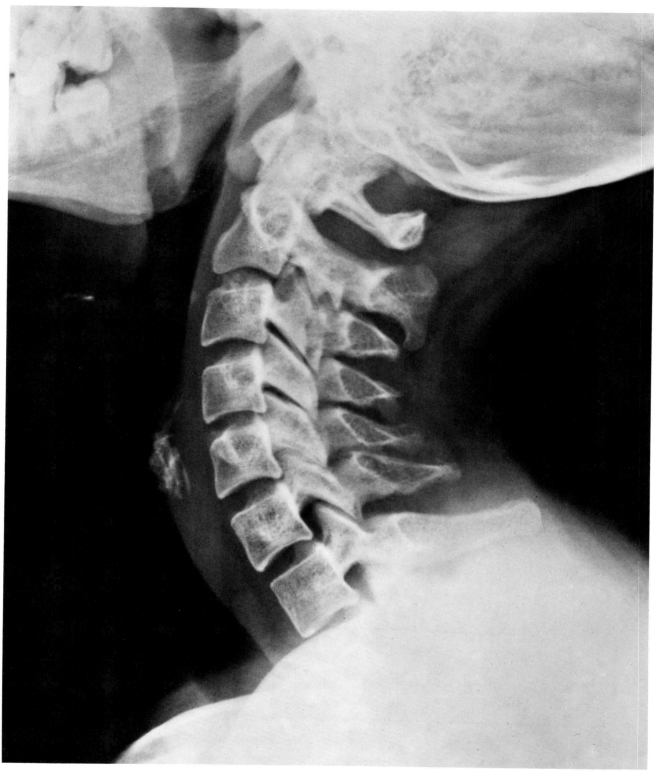

Fig. 56. Cervical spine, lateral view

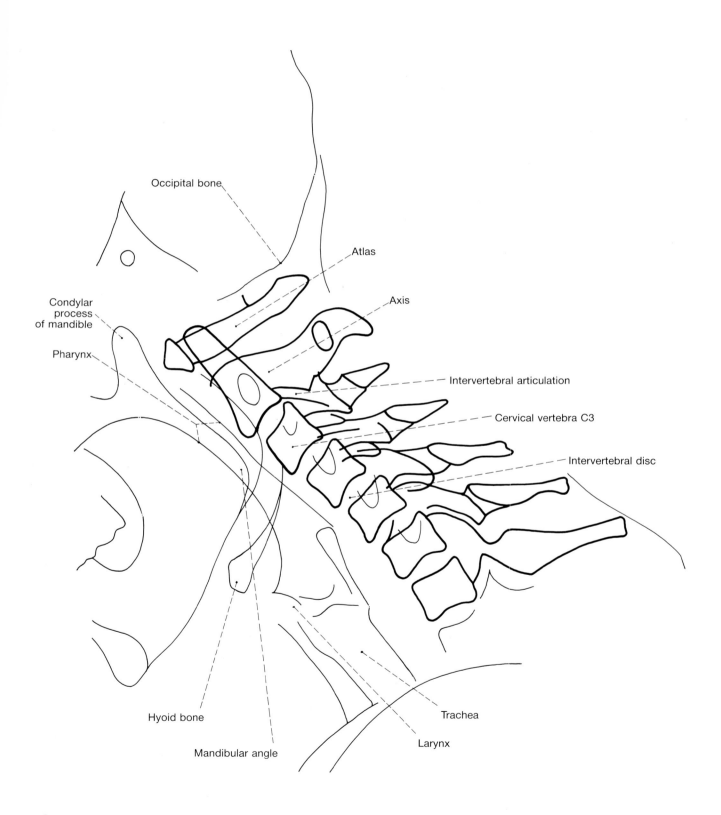

Occipital bone

Atlas

Axis

Condylar
process
of mandible

Pharynx

Intervertebral articulation

Cervical vertebra C3

Intervertebral disc

Hyoid bone

Mandibular angle

Trachea

Larynx

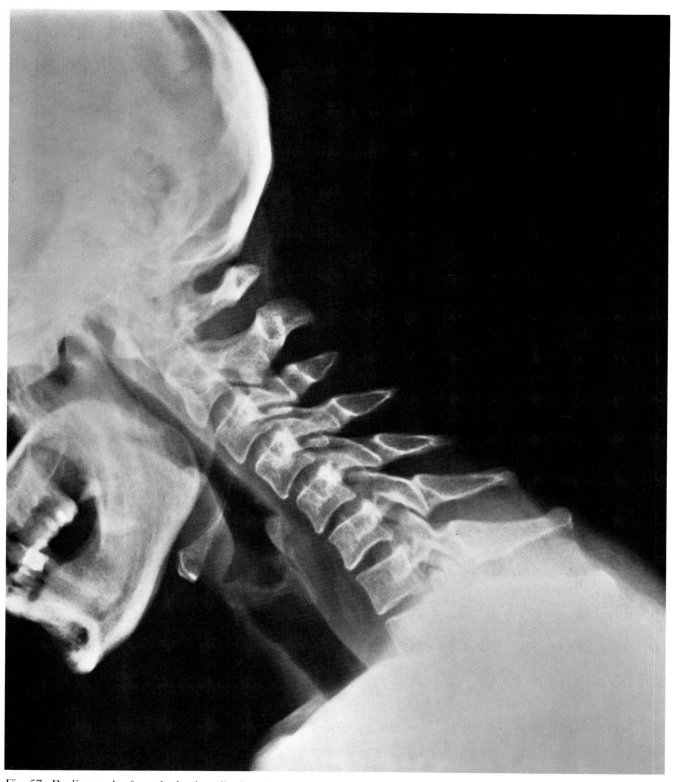

Fig. 57. Radiograph of cervical spine, flexion view

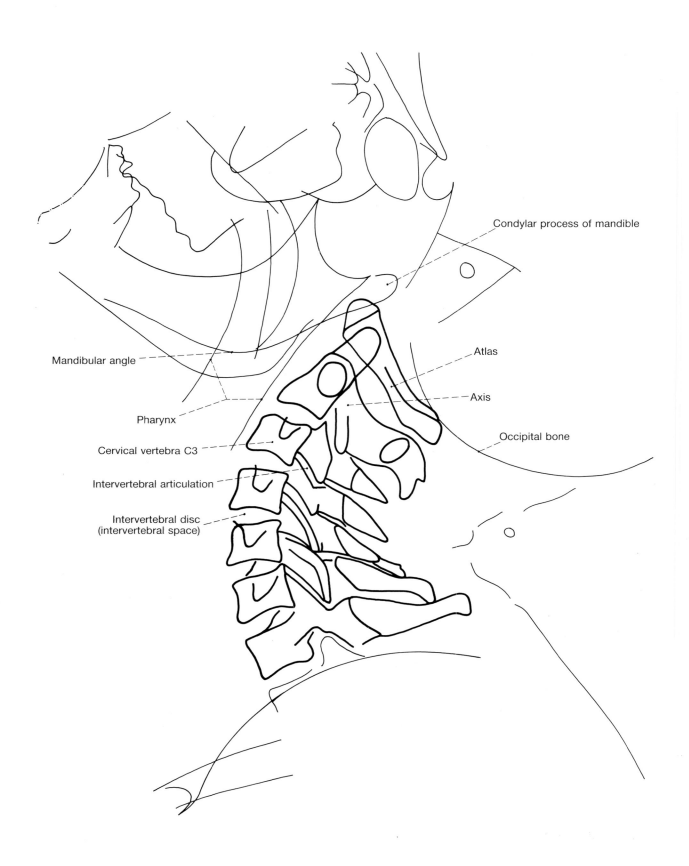

Condylar process of mandible

Atlas

Axis

Occipital bone

Mandibular angle

Pharynx

Cervical vertebra C3

Intervertebral articulation

Intervertebral disc
(intervertebral space)

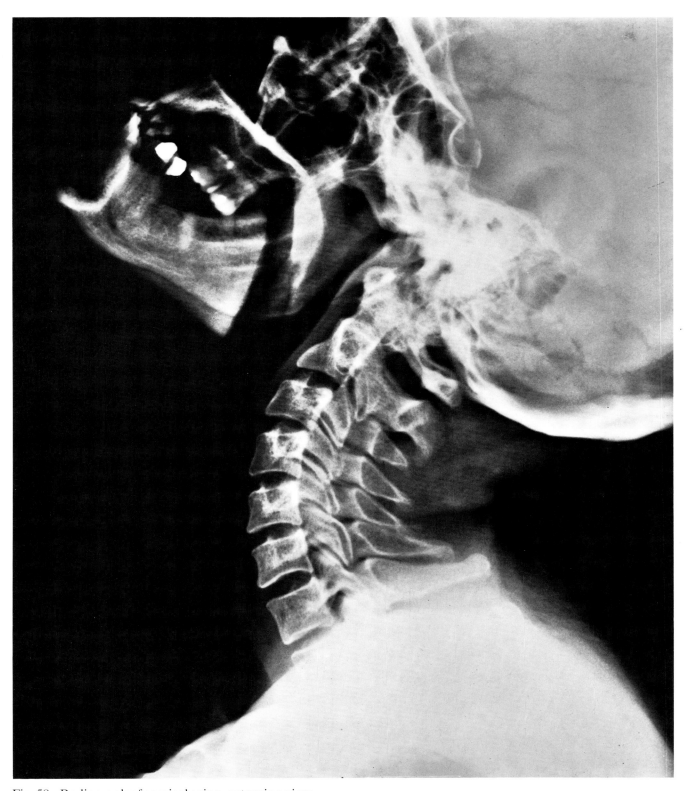

Fig. 58. Radiograph of cervical spine, extension view

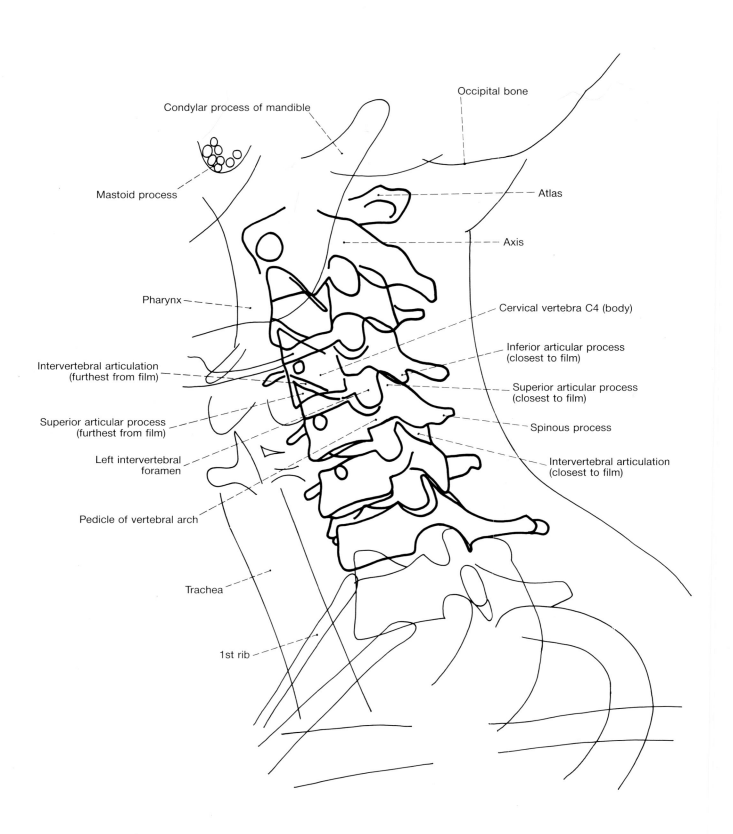

Condylar process of mandible

Occipital bone

Mastoid process

Atlas

Axis

Pharynx

Cervical vertebra C4 (body)

Inferior articular process
(closest to film)

Intervertebral articulation
(furthest from film)

Superior articular process
(closest to film)

Superior articular process
(furthest from film)

Spinous process

Left intervertebral
foramen

Intervertebral articulation
(closest to film)

Pedicle of vertebral arch

Trachea

1st rib

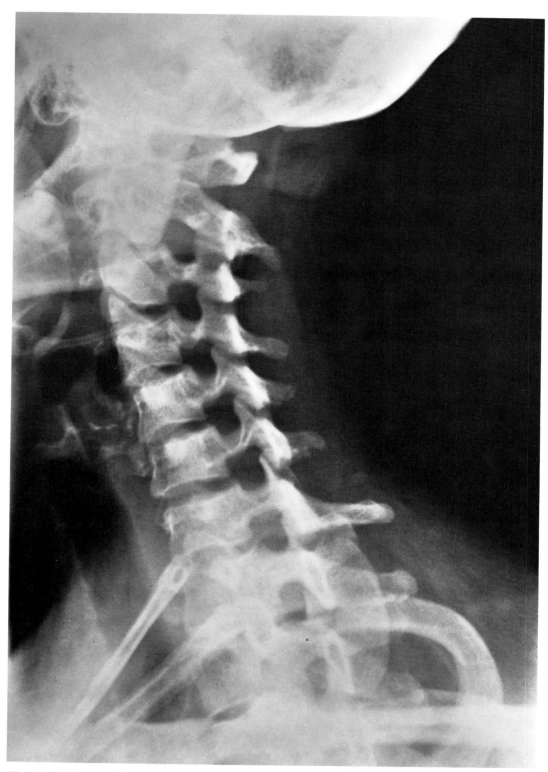

Fig. 59. Oblique radiograph of the cervical spine

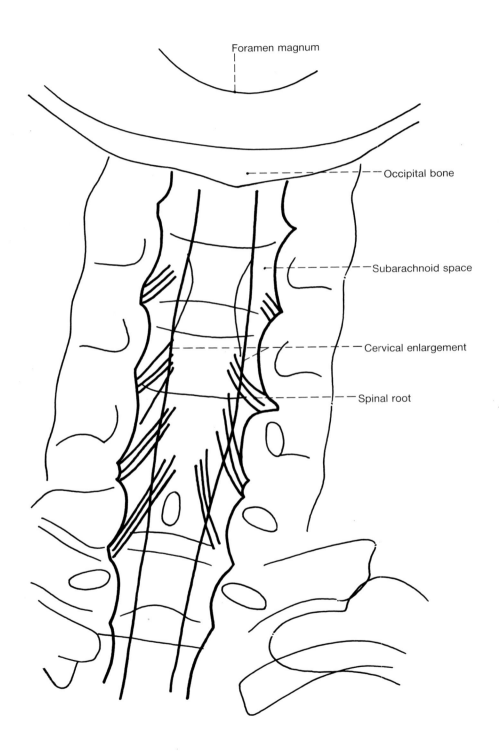

Foramen magnum

Occipital bone

Subarachnoid space

Cervical enlargement

Spinal root

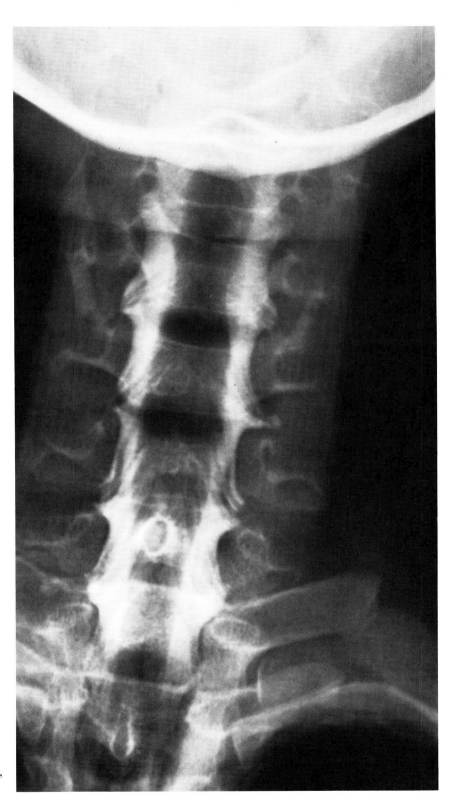

Fig. 60. Cervical myelography,
p.a. view

Thoracic Spine

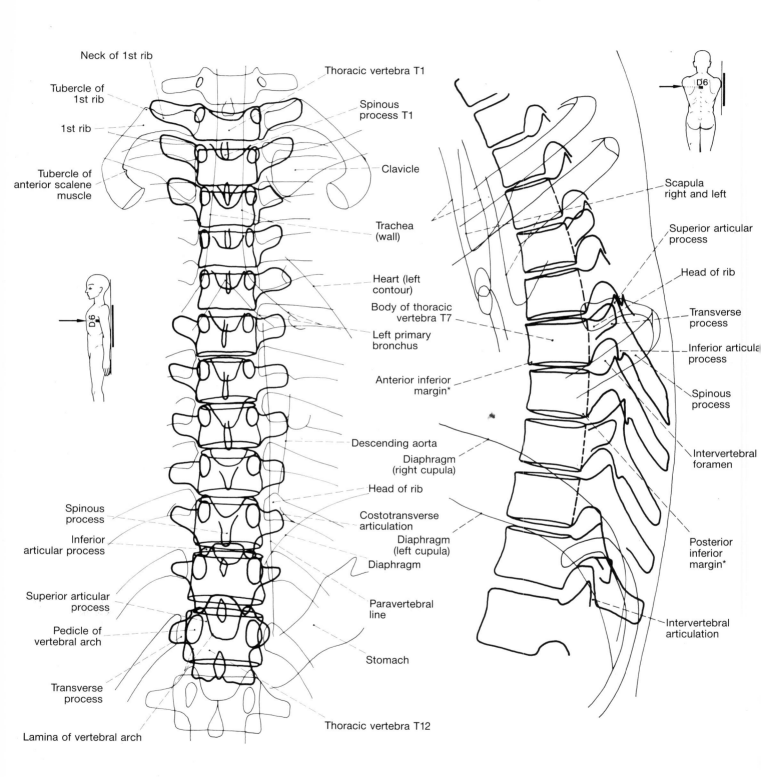

Neck of 1st rib

Tubercle of 1st rib

1st rib

Tubercle of anterior scalene muscle

Thoracic vertebra T1

Spinous process T1

Clavicle

Trachea (wall)

Heart (left contour)

Body of thoracic vertebra T7

Left primary bronchus

Anterior inferior margin*

Descending aorta

Diaphragm (right cupula)

Head of rib

Costotransverse articulation

Diaphragm (left cupula)

Diaphragm

Paravertebral line

Stomach

Thoracic vertebra T12

Spinous process

Inferior articular process

Superior articular process

Pedicle of vertebral arch

Transverse process

Lamina of vertebral arch

Scapula right and left

Superior articular process

Head of rib

Transverse process

Inferior articular process

Spinous process

Intervertebral foramen

Posterior inferior margin*

Intervertebral articulation

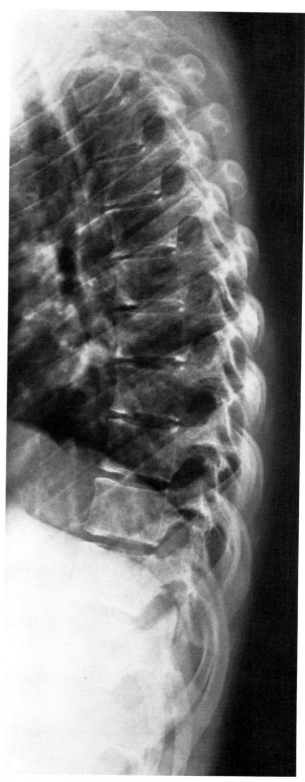

Fig. 61. Thoracic spine, a.p. view   Fig. 62. Thoracic spine, lateral view

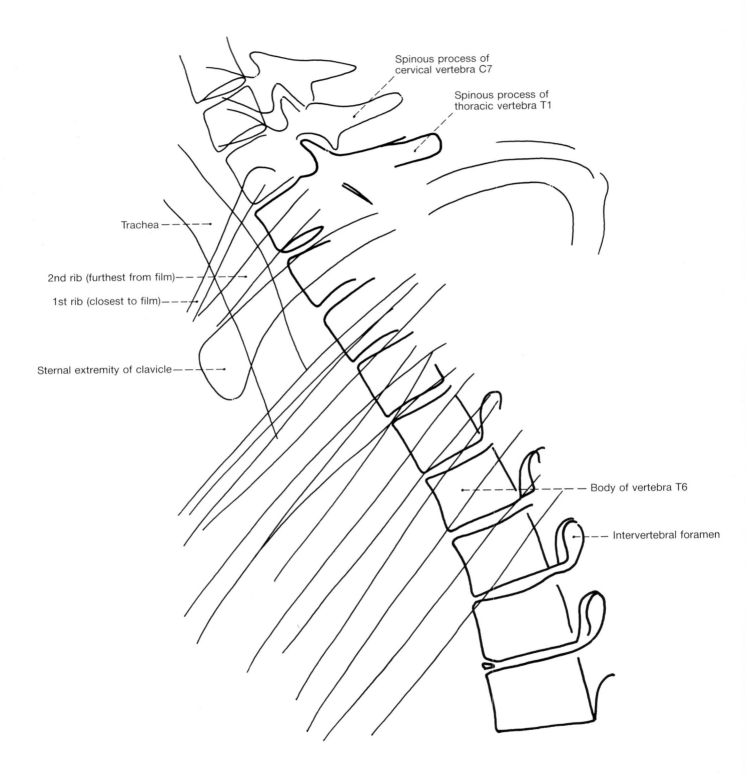

Spinous process of
cervical vertebra C7

Spinous process of
thoracic vertebra T1

Trachea

2nd rib (furthest from film)

1st rib (closest to film)

Sternal extremity of clavicle

Body of vertebra T6

Intervertebral foramen

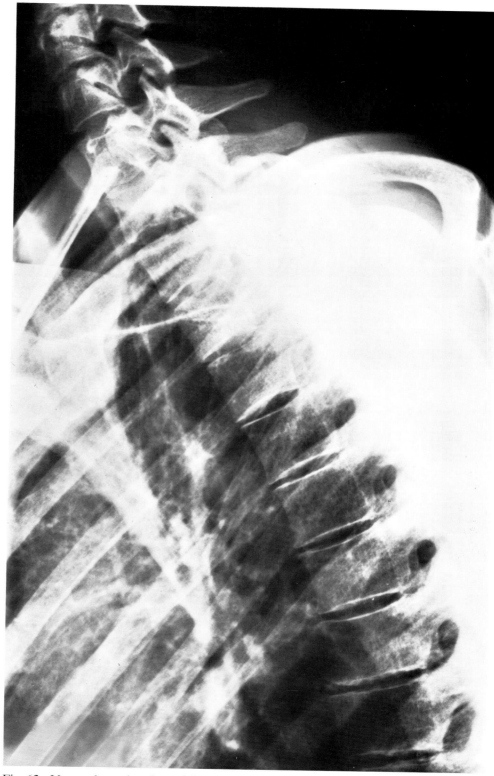

Fig. 63. Upper thoracic spine, oblique view

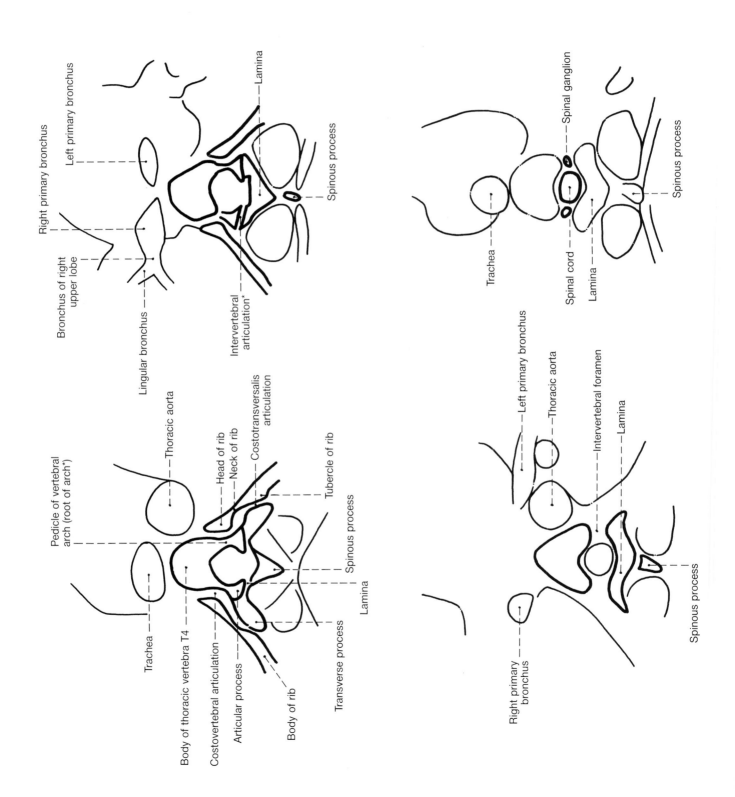

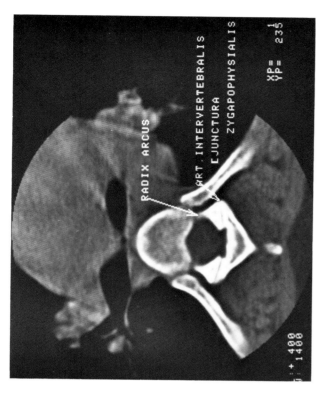

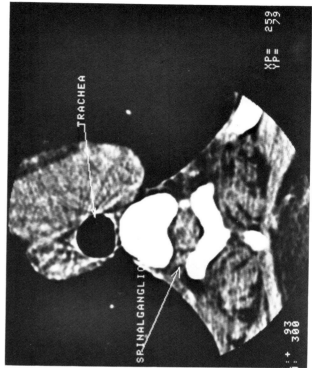

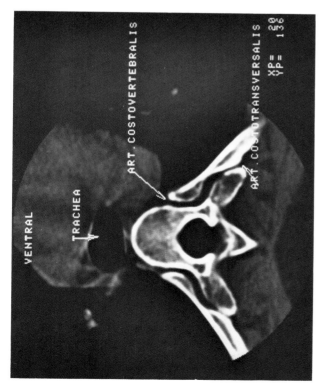

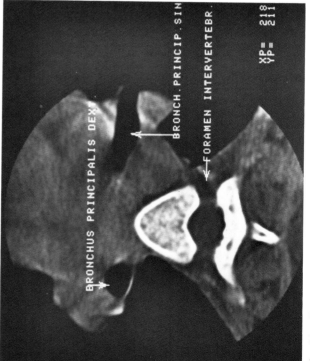

Fig. 64. Computed axial tomograms, T4 to T5

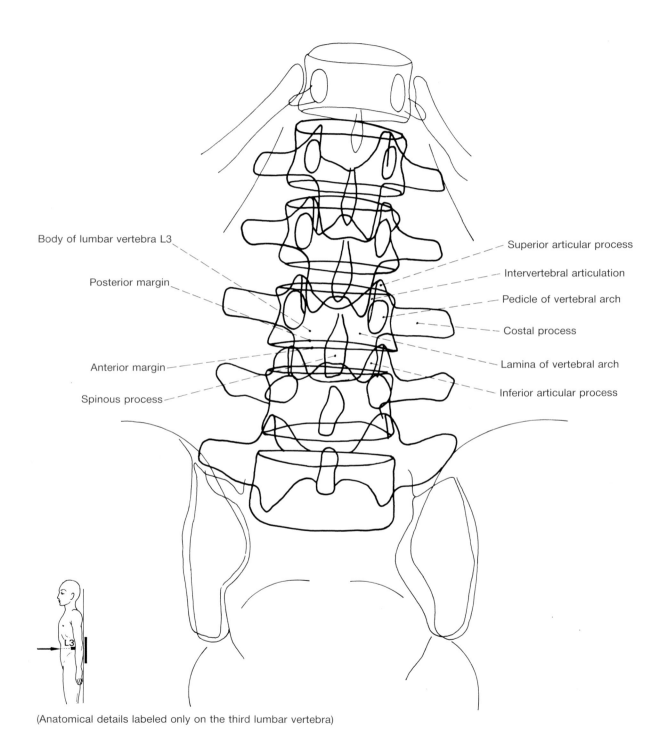

Body of lumbar vertebra L3

Posterior margin

Anterior margin

Spinous process

Superior articular process

Intervertebral articulation

Pedicle of vertebral arch

Costal process

Lamina of vertebral arch

Inferior articular process

L3

(Anatomical details labeled only on the third lumbar vertebra)

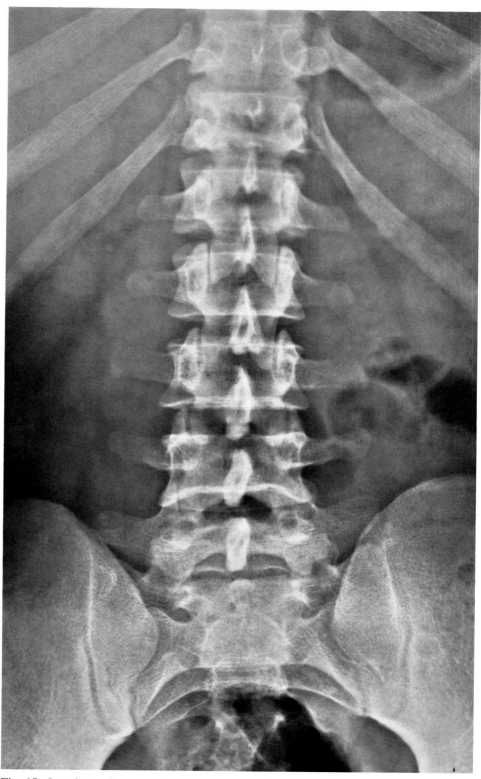

Fig. 65. Lumbar spine, a.p. view

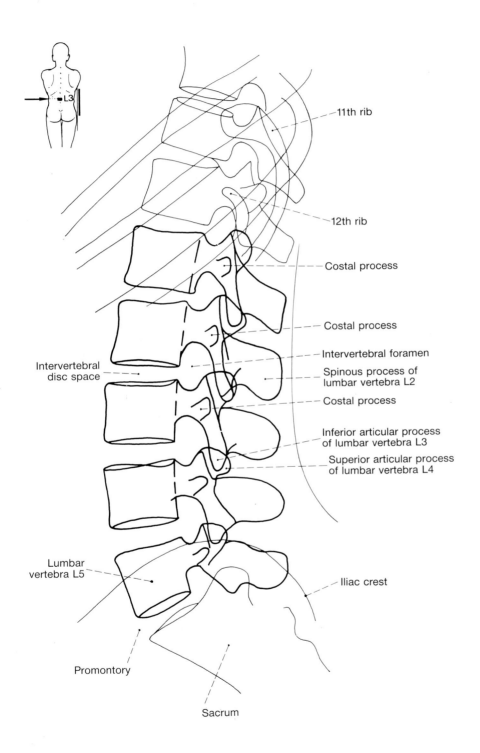

11th rib

12th rib

Costal process

Costal process

Intervertebral foramen

Spinous process of
lumbar vertebra L2

Costal process

Inferior articular process
of lumbar vertebra L3

Superior articular process
of lumbar vertebra L4

Iliac crest

Intervertebral
disc space

Lumbar
vertebra L5

Promontory

Sacrum

L3

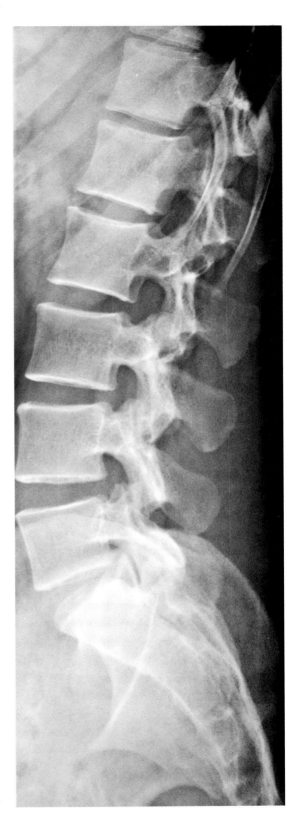

Fig. 66. Lumbar spine, lateral view

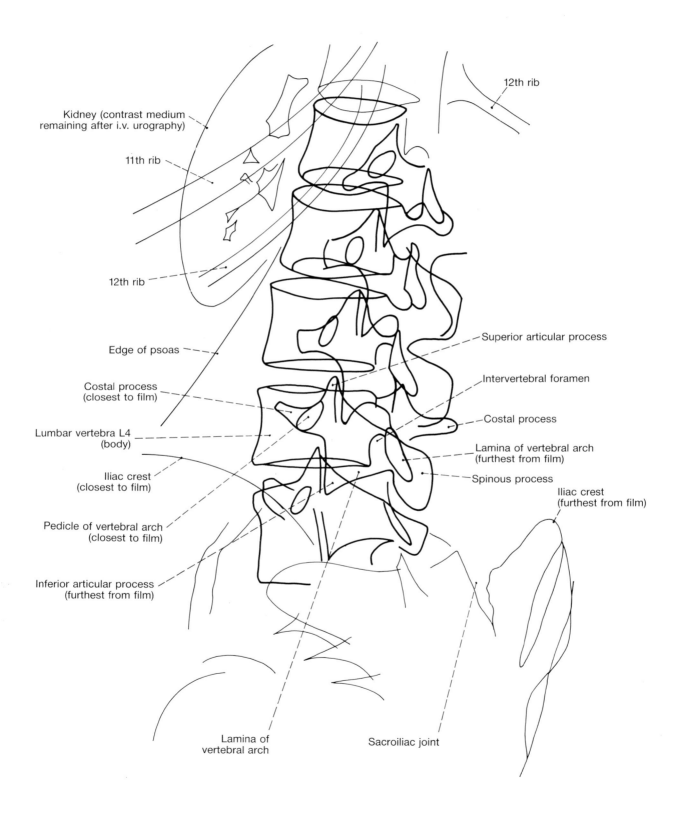

Kidney (contrast medium
remaining after i.v. urography)

11th rib

12th rib

Edge of psoas

Costal process
(closest to film)

Lumbar vertebra L4
(body)

Iliac crest
(closest to film)

Pedicle of vertebral arch
(closest to film)

Inferior articular process
(furthest from film)

12th rib

Superior articular process

Intervertebral foramen

Costal process

Lamina of vertebral arch
(furthest from film)

Spinous process

Iliac crest
(furthest from film)

Lamina of
vertebral arch

Sacroiliac joint

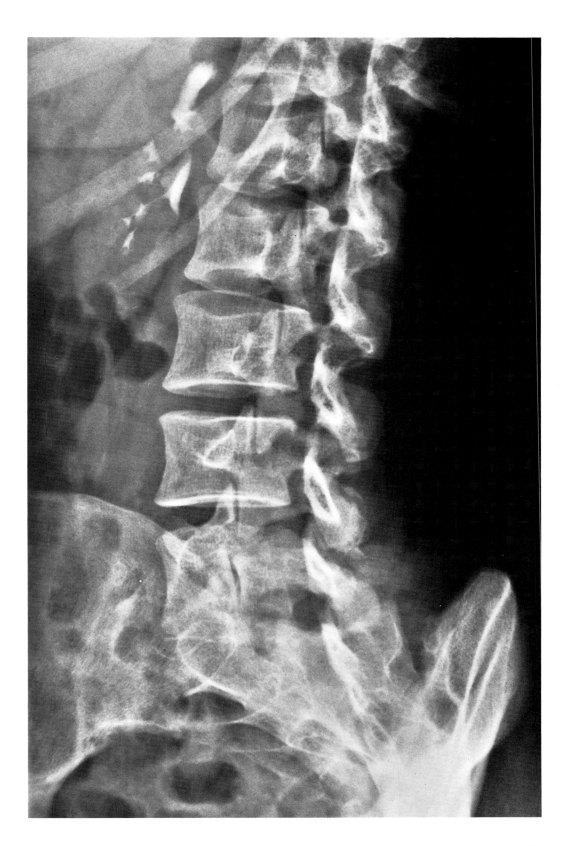

Fig. 67.
Oblique radiograph
of lumbar spine

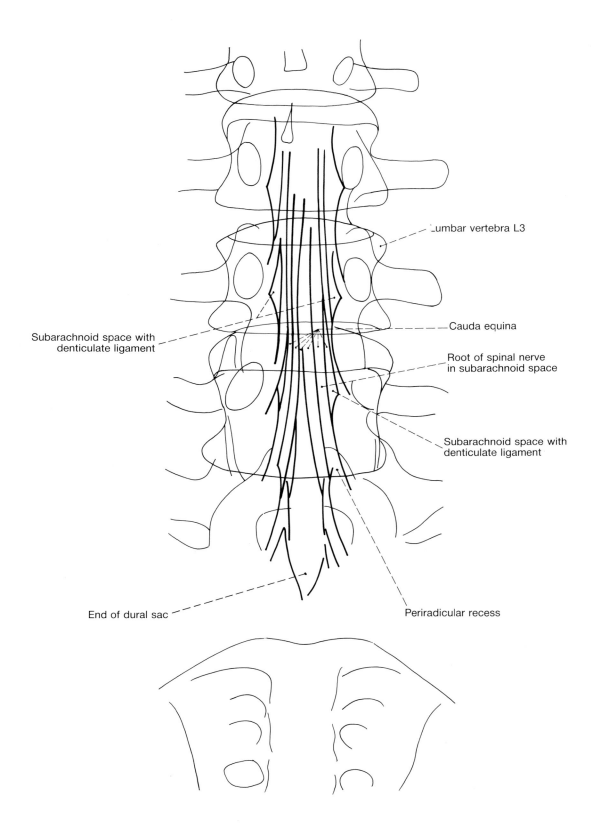

Lumbar vertebra L3

Cauda equina

Subarachnoid space with
denticulate ligament

Root of spinal nerve
in subarachnoid space

Subarachnoid space with
denticulate ligament

End of dural sac

Periradicular recess

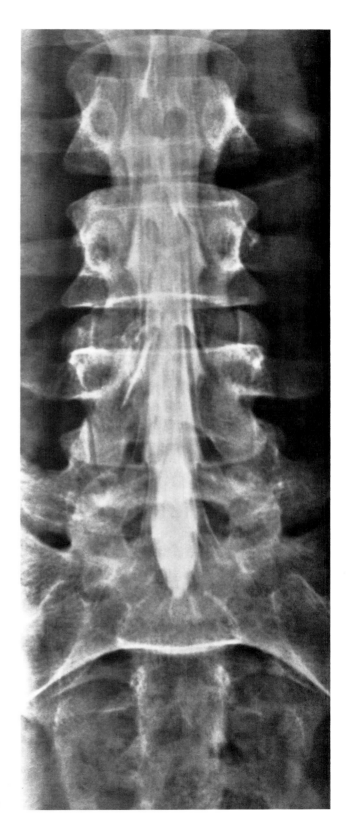

Fig. 68. Myelography, p.a. view

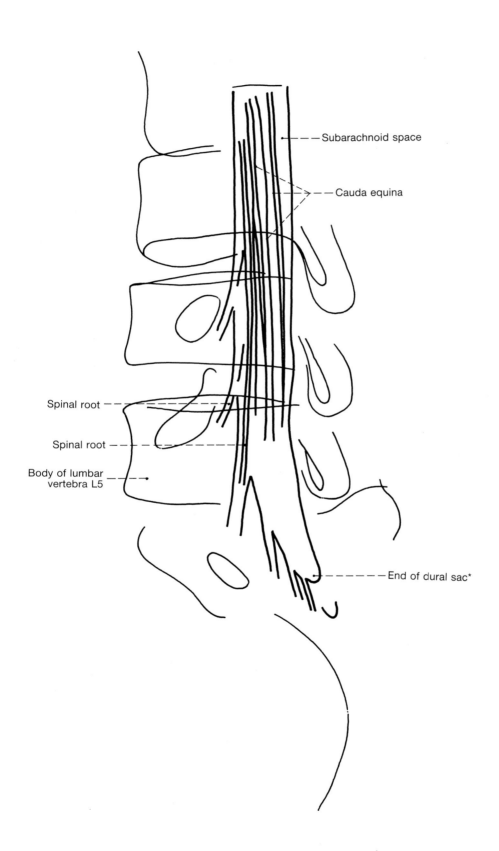

Subarachnoid space

Cauda equina

Spinal root

Spinal root

Body of lumbar
vertebra L5

End of dural sac*

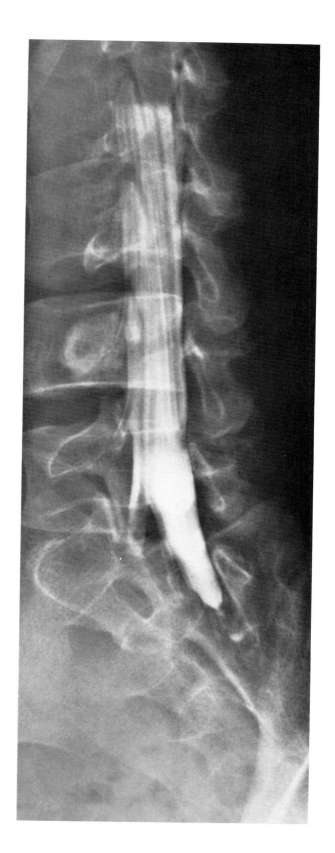

Fig. 69. Lumbar myelography, oblique view

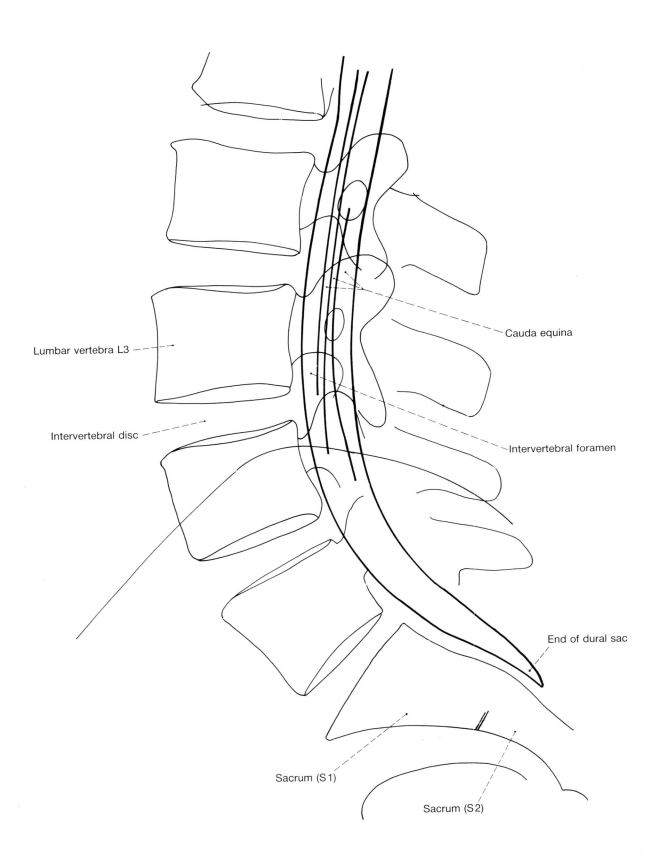

Cauda equina

Lumbar vertebra L3

Intervertebral disc

Intervertebral foramen

End of dural sac

Sacrum (S1)

Sacrum (S2)

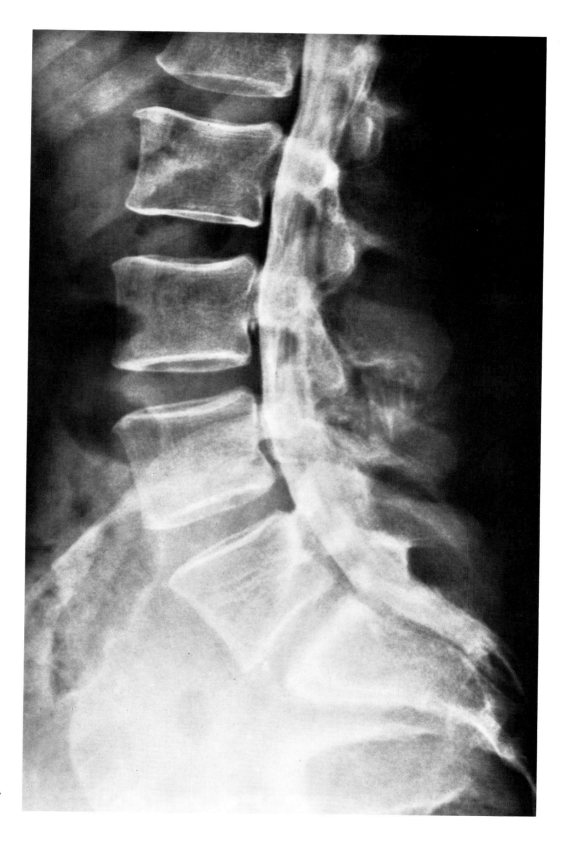

Fig. 70. Myelography,
lateral view

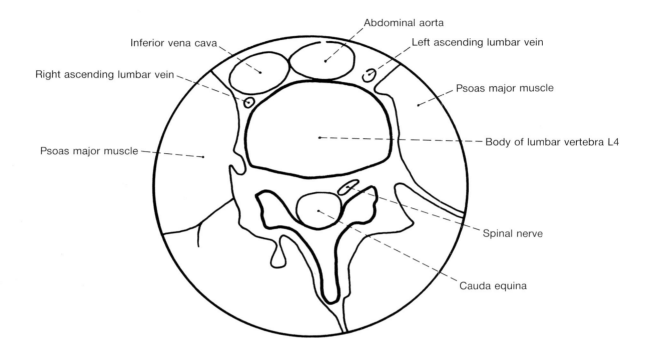

Abdominal aorta

Inferior vena cava

Left ascending lumbar vein

Right ascending lumbar vein

Psoas major muscle

Psoas major muscle

Body of lumbar vertebra L4

Spinal nerve

Cauda equina

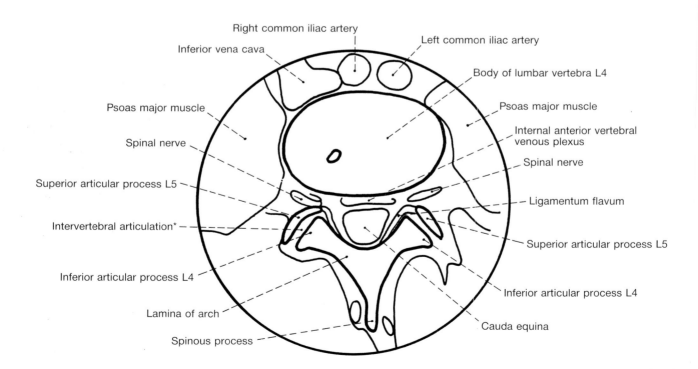

Right common iliac artery

Inferior vena cava

Left common iliac artery

Psoas major muscle

Body of lumbar vertebra L4

Spinal nerve

Psoas major muscle

Superior articular process L5

Internal anterior vertebral venous plexus

Spinal nerve

Intervertebral articulation*

Ligamentum flavum

Inferior articular process L4

Superior articular process L5

Lamina of arch

Inferior articular process L4

Spinous process

Cauda equina

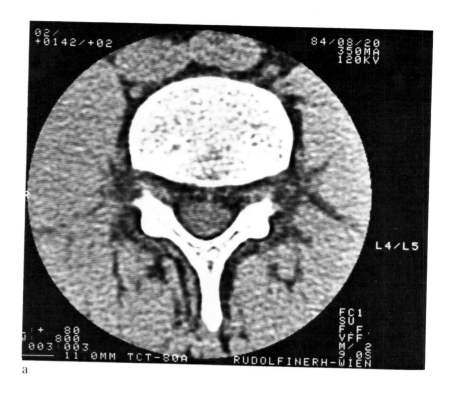

a

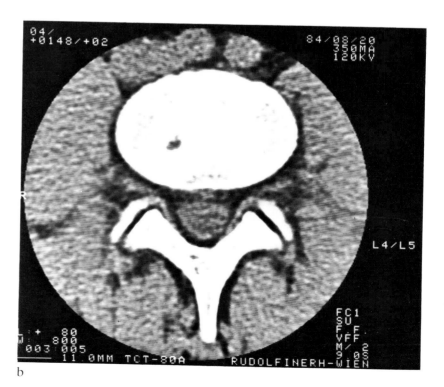

b

Fig. 71a, b.
Computed axial tomograms of
intervertebral disc L4/L5

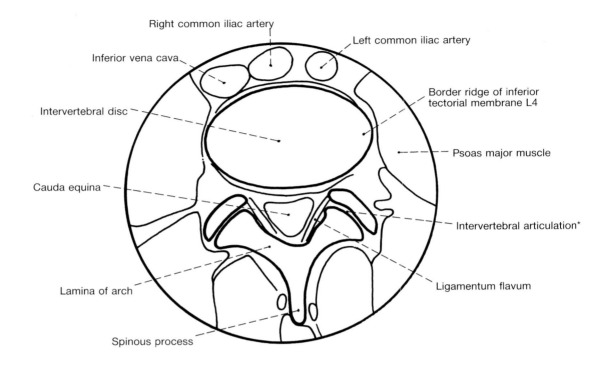

Right common iliac artery

Left common iliac artery

Inferior vena cava

Border ridge of inferior
tectorial membrane L4

Intervertebral disc

Psoas major muscle

Cauda equina

Intervertebral articulation*

Lamina of arch

Ligamentum flavum

Spinous process

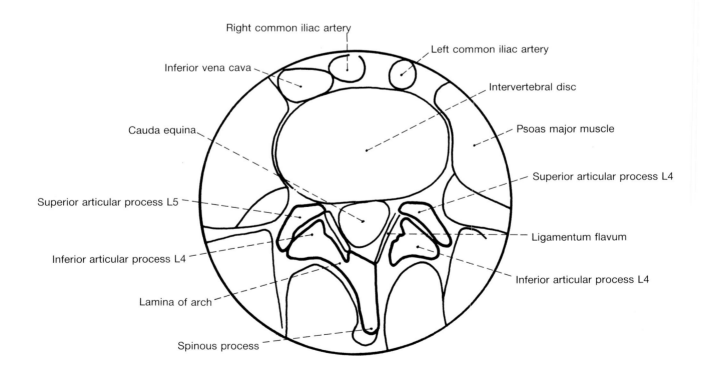

Right common iliac artery

Left common iliac artery

Inferior vena cava

Intervertebral disc

Cauda equina

Psoas major muscle

Superior articular process L4

Superior articular process L5

Inferior articular process L4

Ligamentum flavum

Lamina of arch

Inferior articular process L4

Spinous process

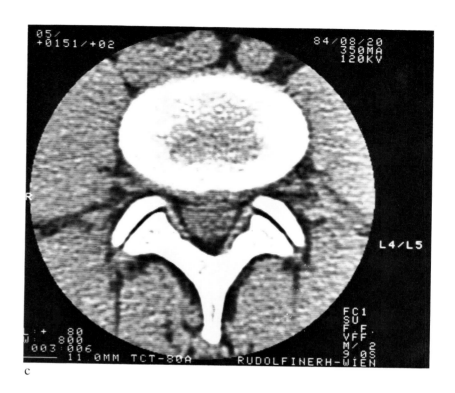

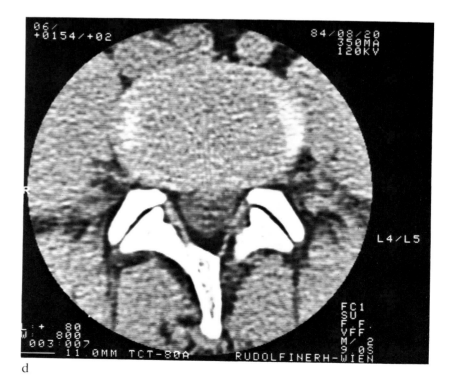

Fig. 71c, d.
Computed axial tomograms of
intervertebral disc L4/L5

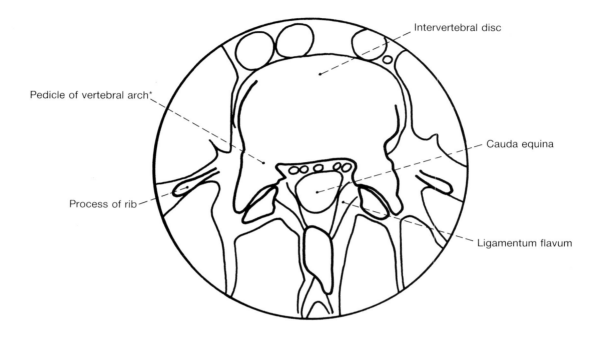

Intervertebral disc

Pedicle of vertebral arch*

Cauda equina

Process of rib

Ligamentum flavum

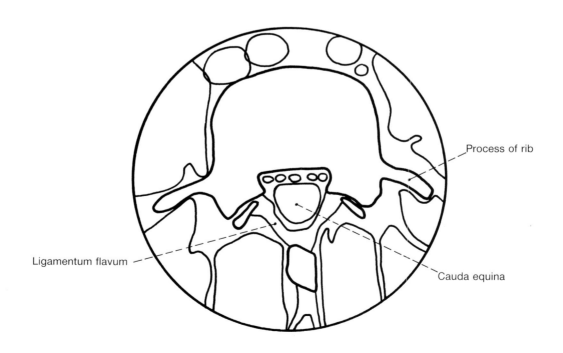

Process of rib

Ligamentum flavum

Cauda equina

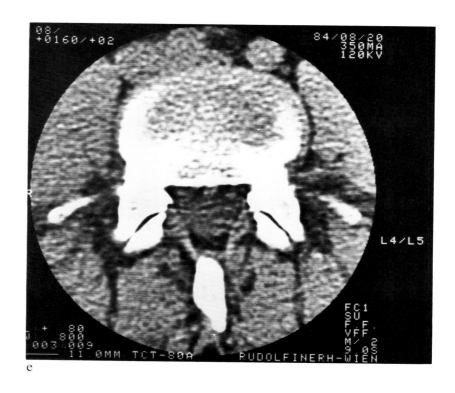

e

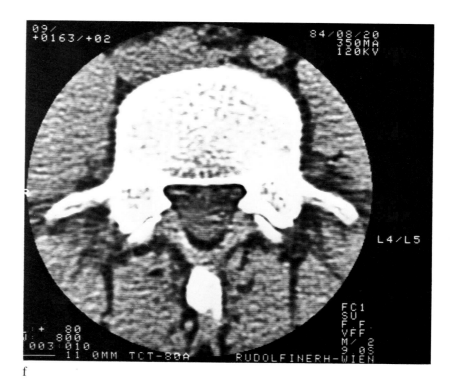

f

Fig. 71 e, f.
Computed axial tomograms of
intervertebral disc L4/L5

Pelvis

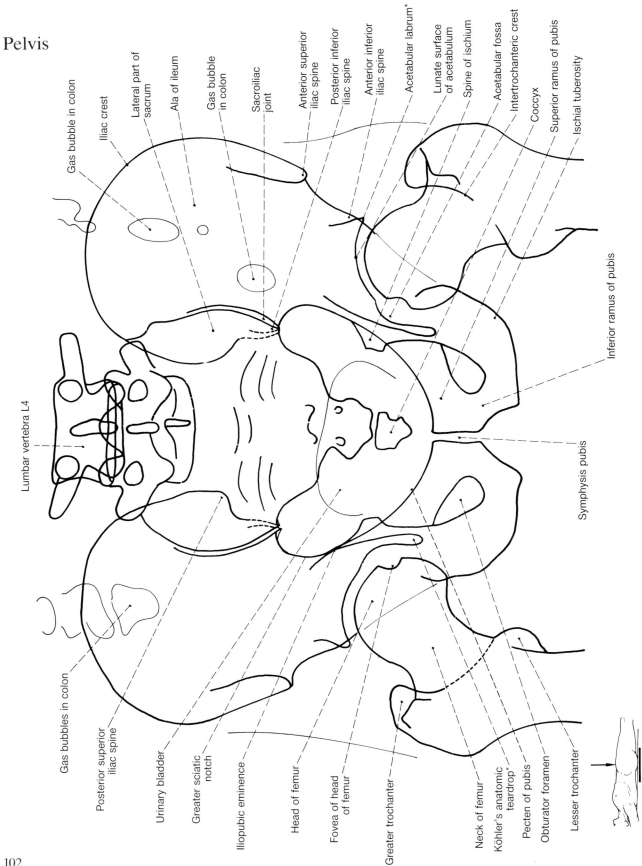

Gas bubble in colon

Iliac crest

Lateral part of sacrum

Ala of ileum

Gas bubble in colon

Sacroiliac joint

Anterior superior iliac spine

Posterior inferior iliac spine

Anterior inferior iliac spine

Acetabular labrum*

Lunate surface of acetabulum

Spine of ischium

Acetabular fossa

Intertrochanteric crest

Coccyx

Superior ramus of pubis

Ischial tuberosity

Inferior ramus of pubis

Lumbar vertebra L4

Symphysis pubis

Gas bubbles in colon

Posterior superior iliac spine

Urinary bladder

Greater sciatic notch

Iliopubic eminence

Head of femur

Fovea of head of femur

Greater trochanter

Neck of femur

Köhler's anatomic teardrop*

Pecten of pubis

Obturator foramen

Lesser trochanter

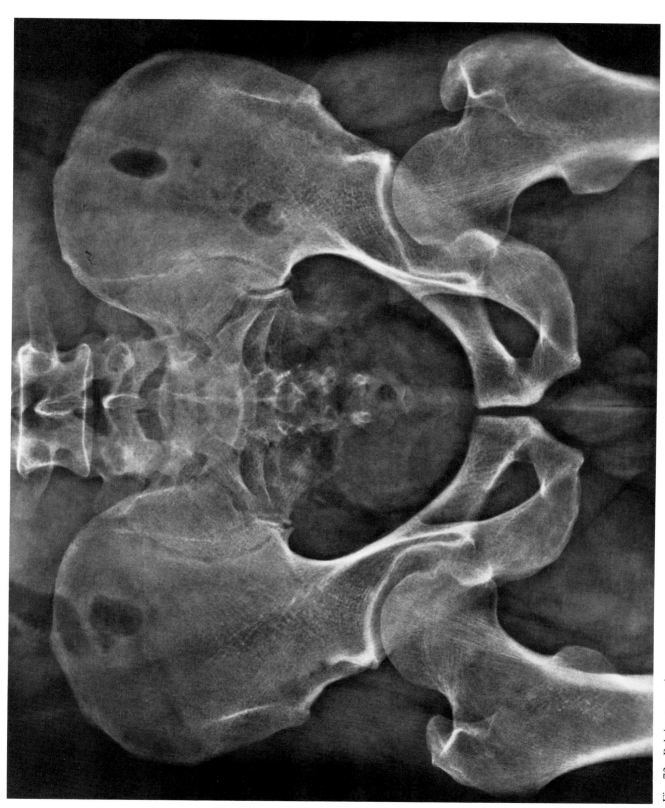

Fig. 72. Pelvis, a.p. view

Sacrum and Coccyx

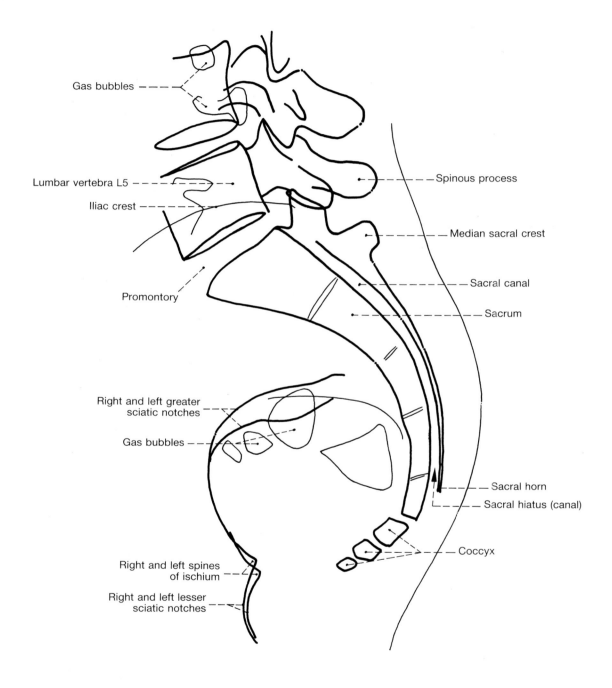

Gas bubbles

Lumbar vertebra L5

Iliac crest

Promontory

Right and left greater
sciatic notches

Gas bubbles

Right and left spines
of ischium

Right and left lesser
sciatic notches

Spinous process

Median sacral crest

Sacral canal

Sacrum

Sacral horn

Sacral hiatus (canal)

Coccyx

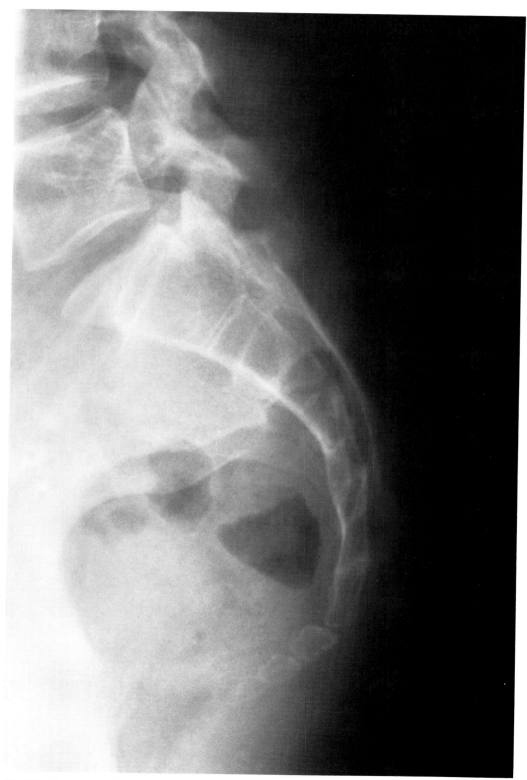

Fig. 73. Sacrum and coccyx, lateral view

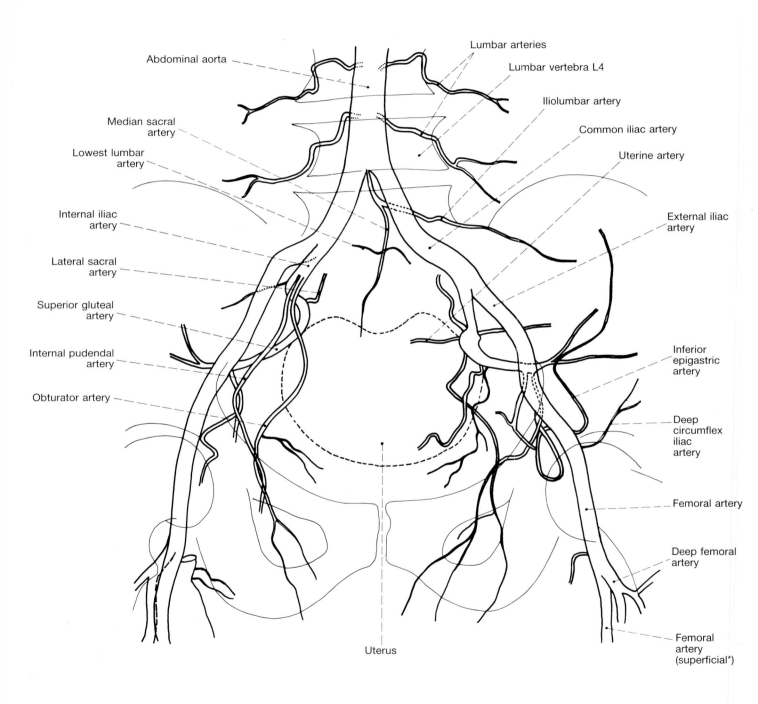

Abdominal aorta

Lumbar arteries

Lumbar vertebra L4

Median sacral
artery

Iliolumbar artery

Common iliac artery

Lowest lumbar
artery

Uterine artery

Internal iliac
artery

External iliac
artery

Lateral sacral
artery

Superior gluteal
artery

Inferior
epigastric
artery

Internal pudendal
artery

Obturator artery

Deep
circumflex
iliac
artery

Femoral artery

Deep femoral
artery

Femoral
artery
(superficial*)

Uterus

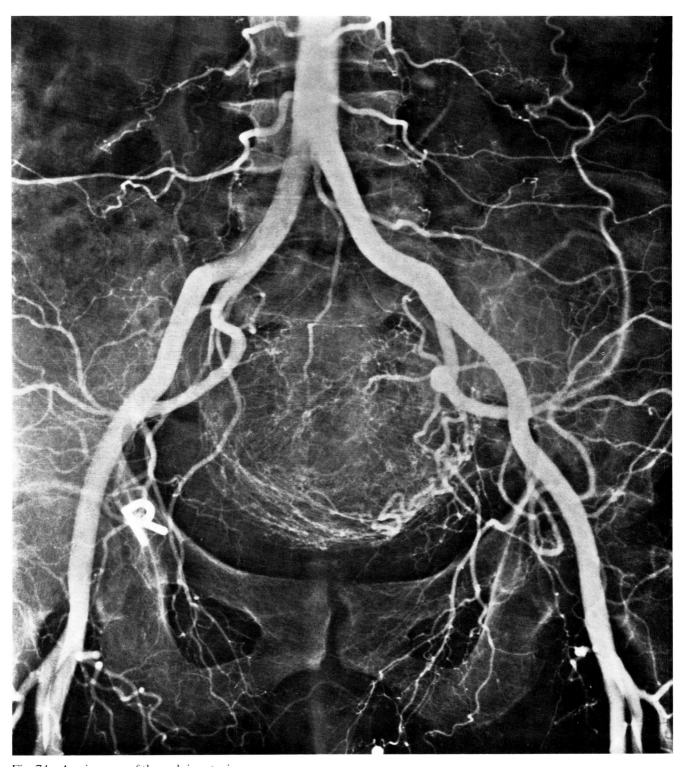

Fig. 74. Angiogram of the pelvic arteries

Upper Extremity

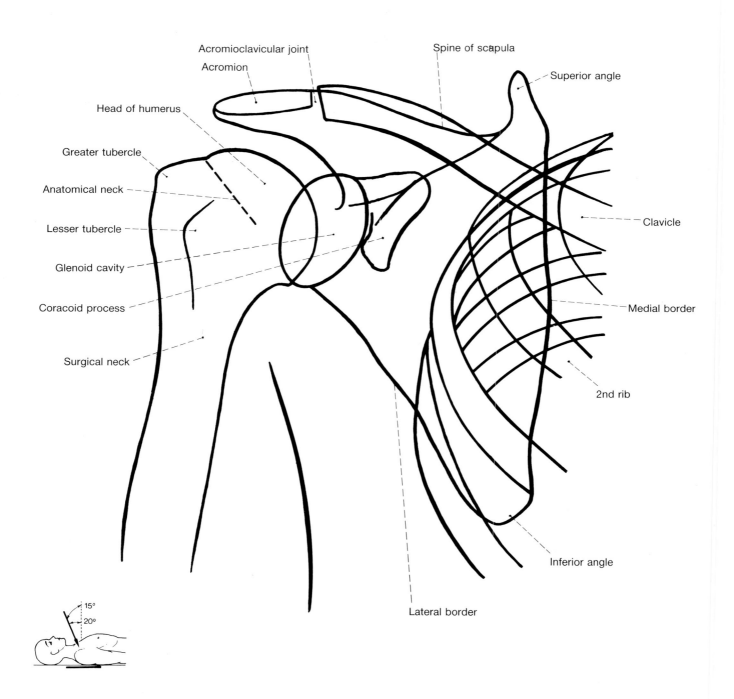

Acromioclavicular joint

Spine of scapula

Acromion

Superior angle

Head of humerus

Greater tubercle

Clavicle

Anatomical neck

Lesser tubercle

Glenoid cavity

Medial border

Coracoid process

Surgical neck

2nd rib

Lateral border

Inferior angle

15°
20°

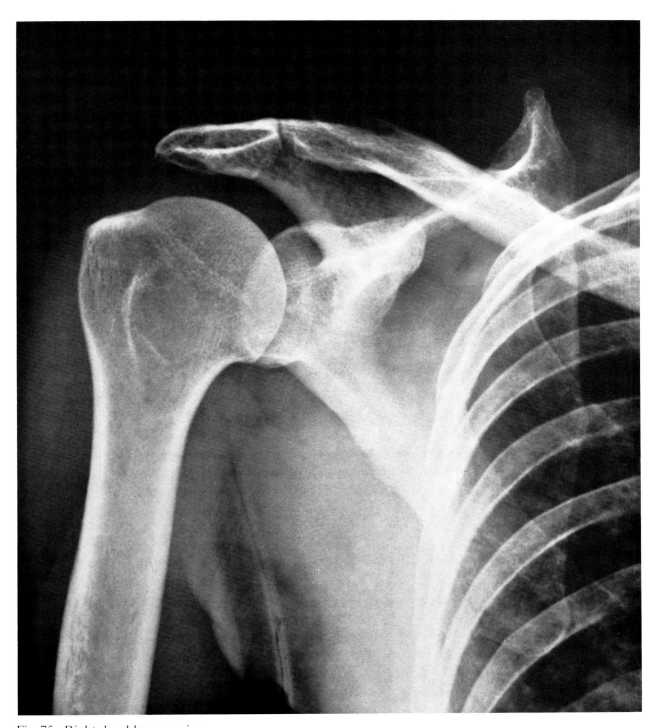

Fig. 75. Right shoulder, a.p. view

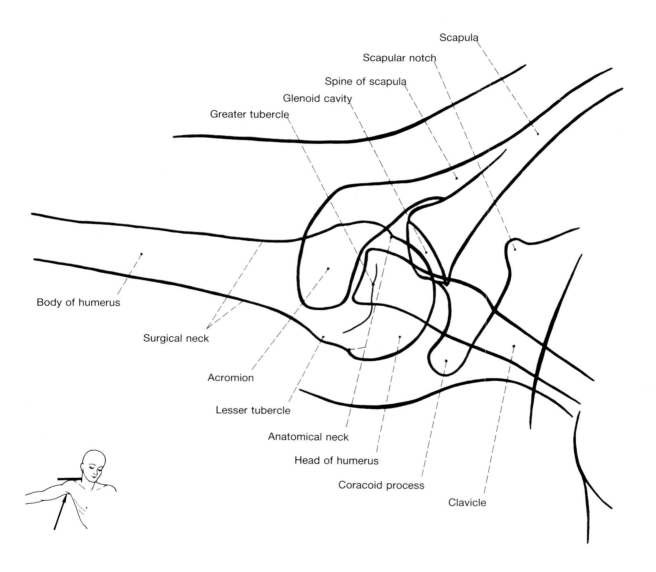

Scapula

Scapular notch

Spine of scapula

Glenoid cavity

Greater tubercle

Body of humerus

Surgical neck

Acromion

Lesser tubercle

Anatomical neck

Head of humerus

Coracoid process

Clavicle

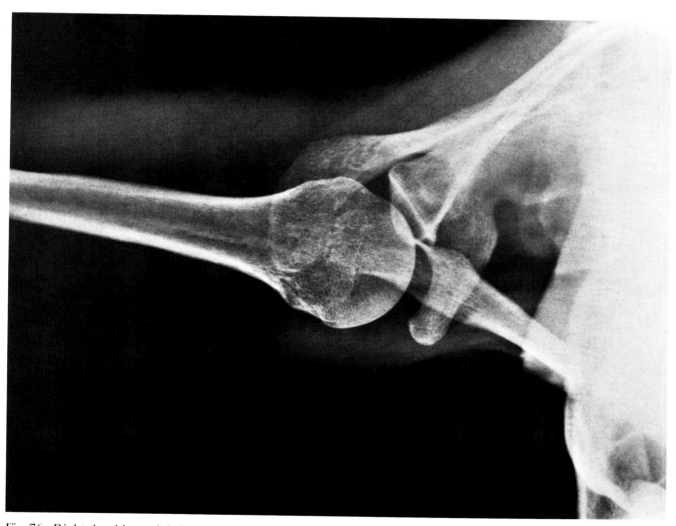

Fig. 76. Right shoulder, axial view

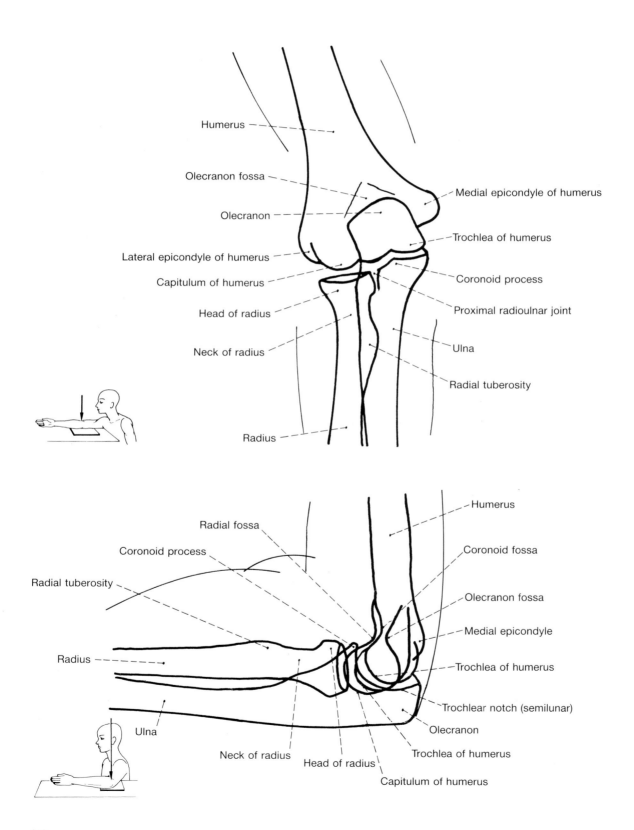

Humerus

Olecranon fossa

Olecranon

Lateral epicondyle of humerus

Capitulum of humerus

Head of radius

Neck of radius

Radius

Medial epicondyle of humerus

Trochlea of humerus

Coronoid process

Proximal radioulnar joint

Ulna

Radial tuberosity

Radial fossa

Coronoid process

Radial tuberosity

Radius

Ulna

Neck of radius

Head of radius

Humerus

Coronoid fossa

Olecranon fossa

Medial epicondyle

Trochlea of humerus

Trochlear notch (semilunar)

Olecranon

Trochlea of humerus

Capitulum of humerus

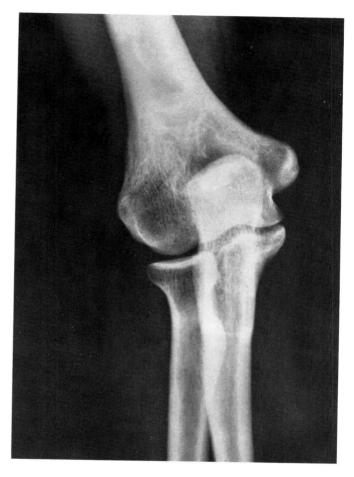

Fig. 77. Right elbow, a.p. view

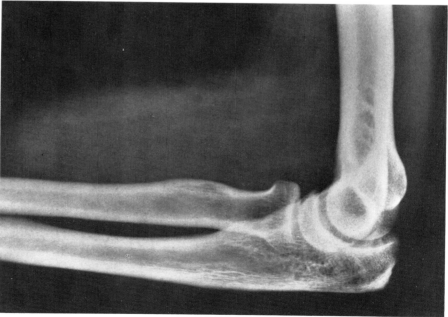

Fig. 78. Left elbow,
lateral view

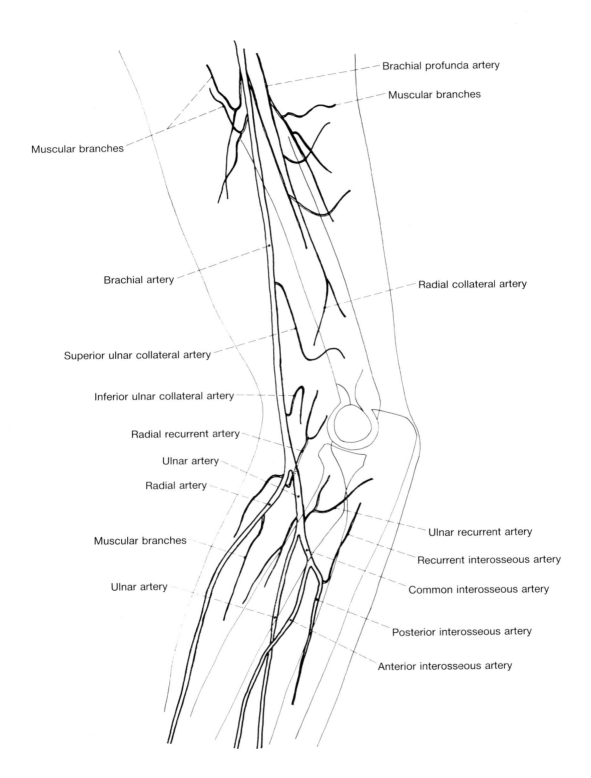

Brachial profunda artery

Muscular branches

Muscular branches

Brachial artery

Radial collateral artery

Superior ulnar collateral artery

Inferior ulnar collateral artery

Radial recurrent artery

Ulnar artery

Radial artery

Muscular branches

Ulnar recurrent artery

Recurrent interosseous artery

Common interosseous artery

Ulnar artery

Posterior interosseous artery

Anterior interosseous artery

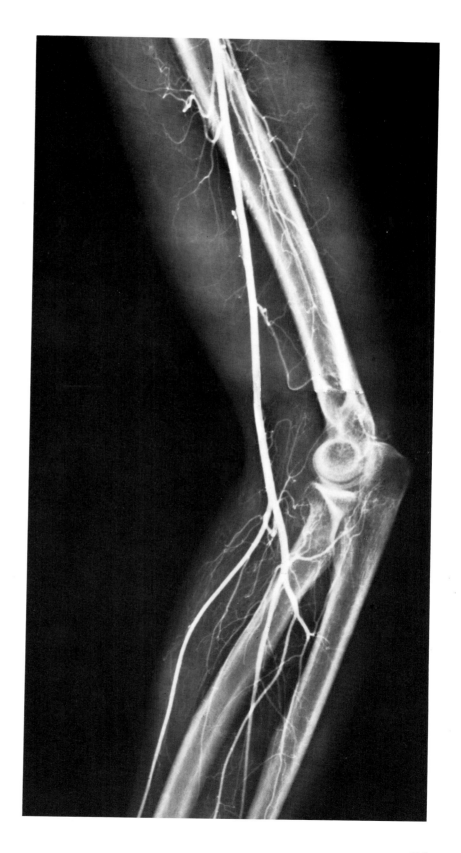

Fig. 79. Angiogram of the elbow

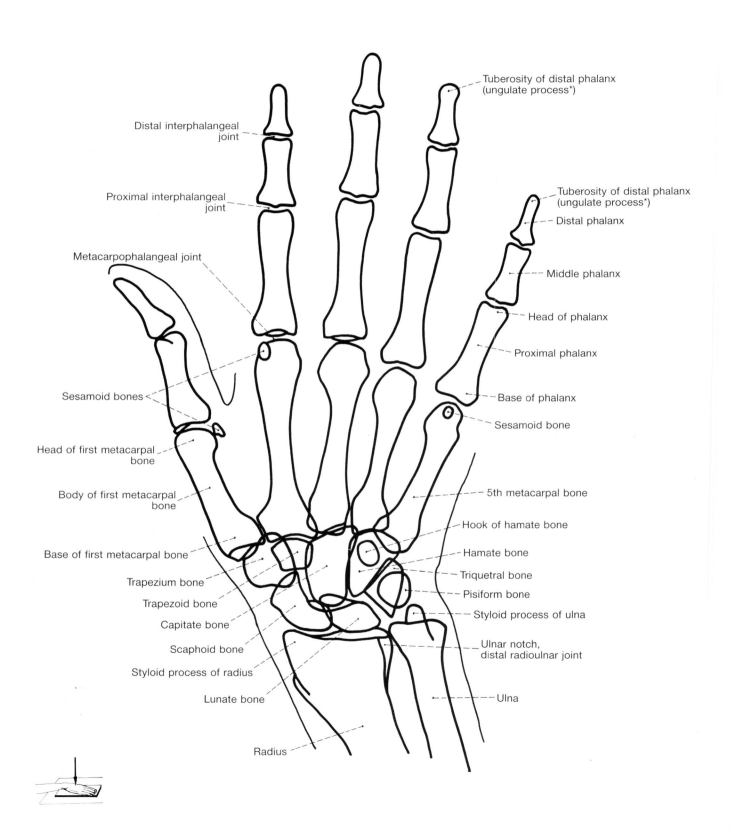

Tuberosity of distal phalanx
(ungulate process*)

Distal interphalangeal
joint

Proximal interphalangeal
joint

Metacarpophalangeal joint

Tuberosity of distal phalanx
(ungulate process*)

Distal phalanx

Middle phalanx

Head of phalanx

Proximal phalanx

Base of phalanx

Sesamoid bones

Head of first metacarpal
bone

Body of first metacarpal
bone

Sesamoid bone

5th metacarpal bone

Hook of hamate bone

Base of first metacarpal bone

Trapezium bone

Trapezoid bone

Capitate bone

Scaphoid bone

Styloid process of radius

Lunate bone

Hamate bone

Triquetral bone

Pisiform bone

Styloid process of ulna

Ulnar notch,
distal radioulnar joint

Ulna

Radius

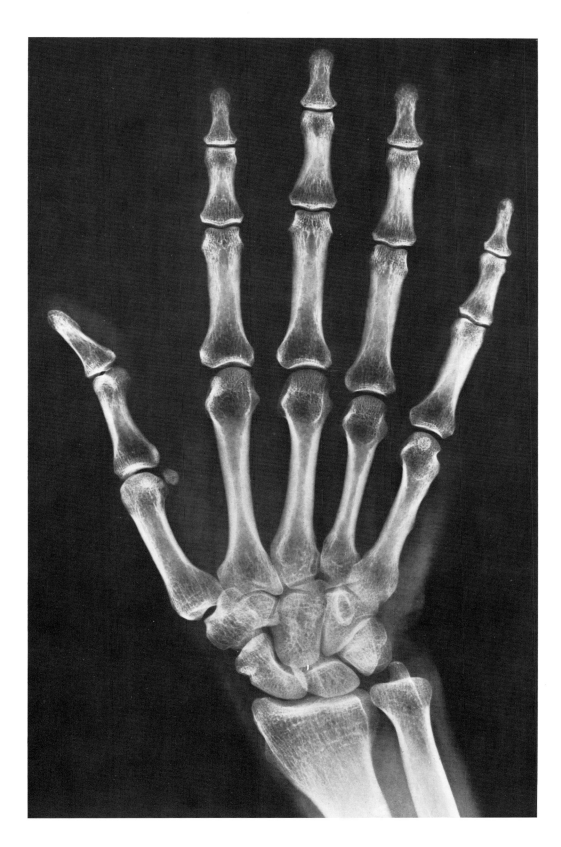

Fig. 80. Right hand,
dorsovolar (palmar)
view

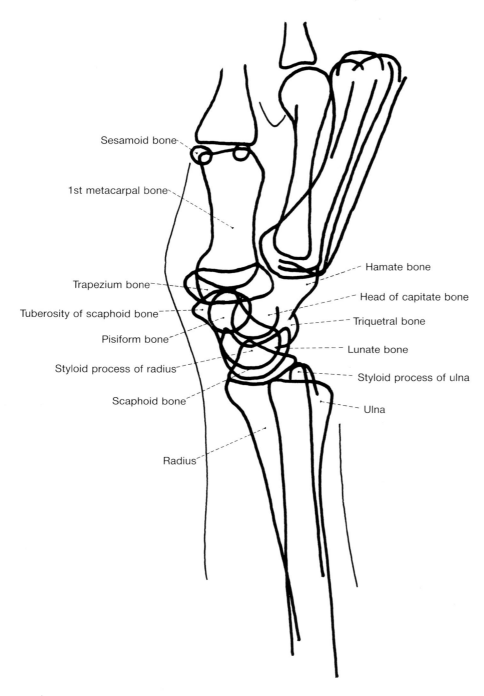

Sesamoid bone

1st metacarpal bone

Trapezium bone

Tuberosity of scaphoid bone

Pisiform bone

Styloid process of radius

Scaphoid bone

Radius

Hamate bone

Head of capitate bone

Triquetral bone

Lunate bone

Styloid process of ulna

Ulna

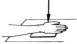

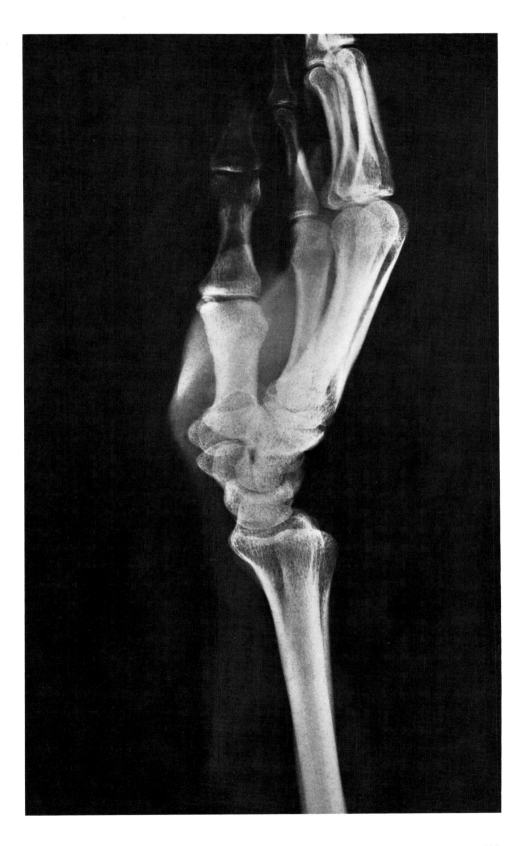

Fig. 81. Right hand,
lateral view

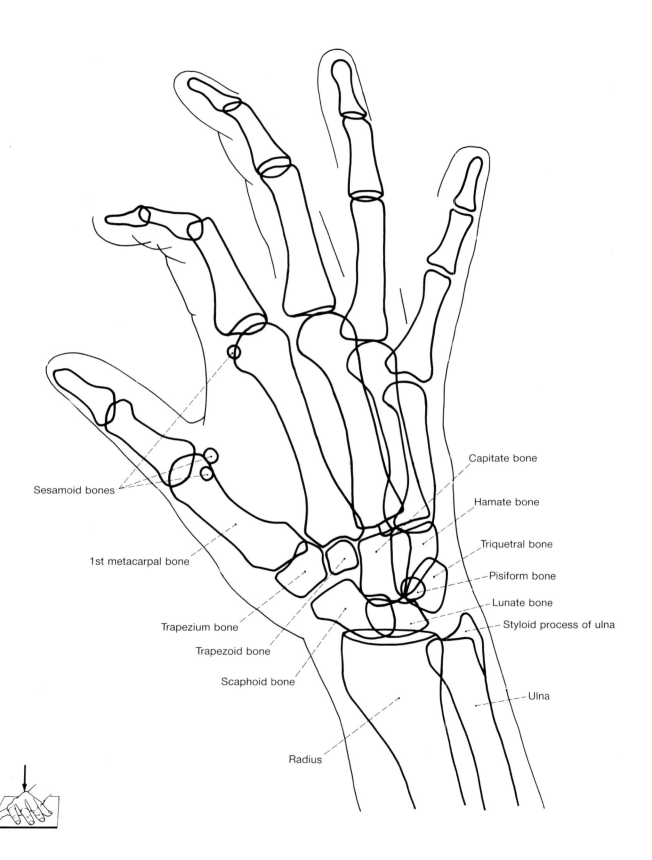

Capitate bone

Hamate bone

Triquetral bone

Pisiform bone

Sesamoid bones

Lunate bone

Styloid process of ulna

1st metacarpal bone

Trapezium bone

Ulna

Trapezoid bone

Scaphoid bone

Radius

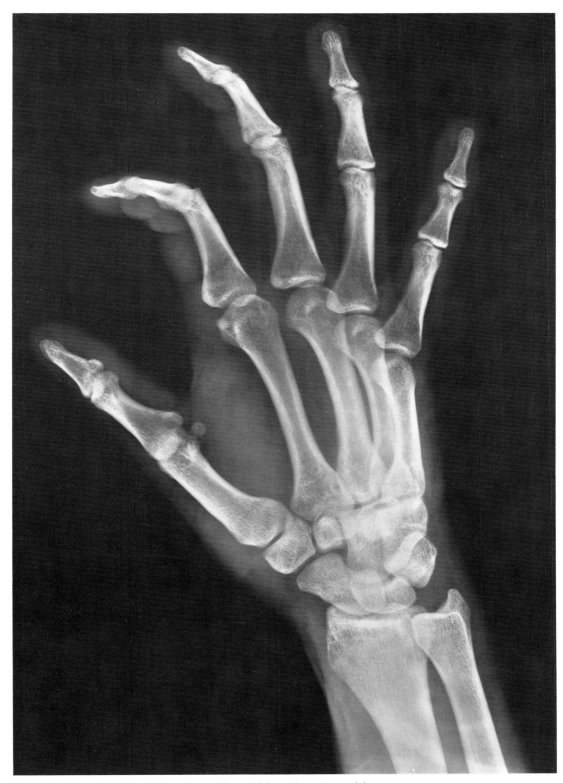

Fig. 82. Right hand, lateral oblique view, Zither player's position

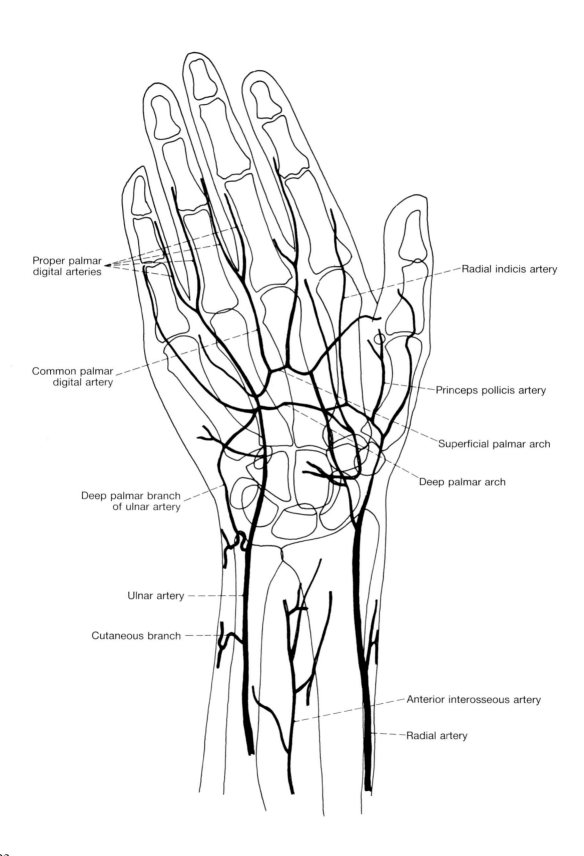

Proper palmar
digital arteries

Radial indicis artery

Common palmar
digital artery

Princeps pollicis artery

Superficial palmar arch

Deep palmar arch

Deep palmar branch
of ulnar artery

Ulnar artery

Cutaneous branch

Anterior interosseous artery

Radial artery

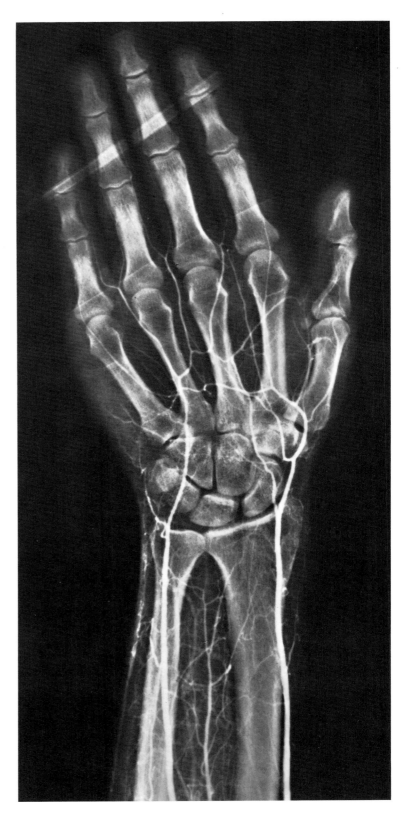

Fig. 83. Angiogram of the hand

Lower Extremity

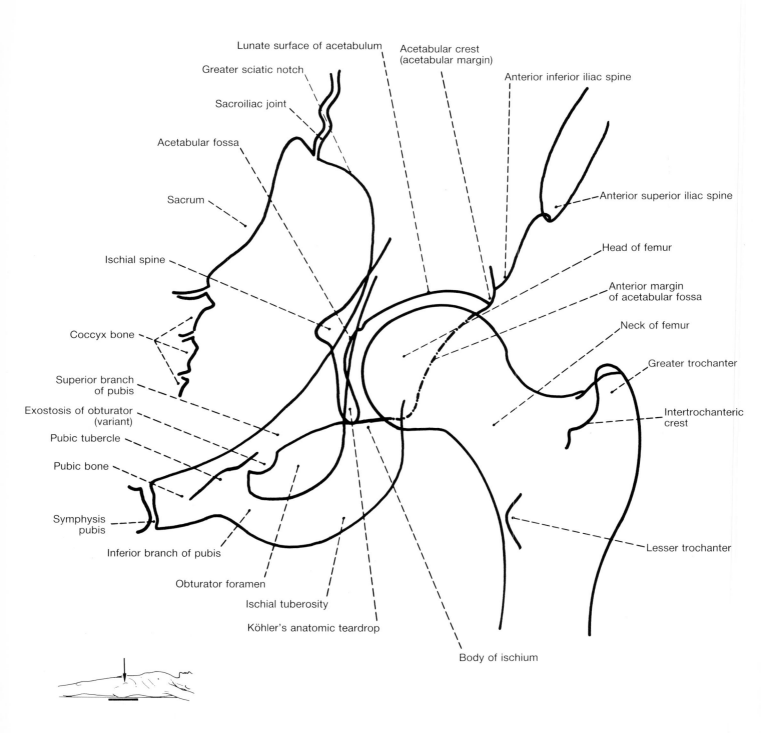

Lunate surface of acetabulum

Greater sciatic notch

Acetabular crest (acetabular margin)

Anterior inferior iliac spine

Sacroiliac joint

Acetabular fossa

Anterior superior iliac spine

Sacrum

Ischial spine

Head of femur

Anterior margin of acetabular fossa

Neck of femur

Coccyx bone

Greater trochanter

Superior branch of pubis

Intertrochanteric crest

Exostosis of obturator (variant)

Pubic tubercle

Pubic bone

Symphysis pubis

Inferior branch of pubis

Lesser trochanter

Obturator foramen

Ischial tuberosity

Köhler's anatomic teardrop

Body of ischium

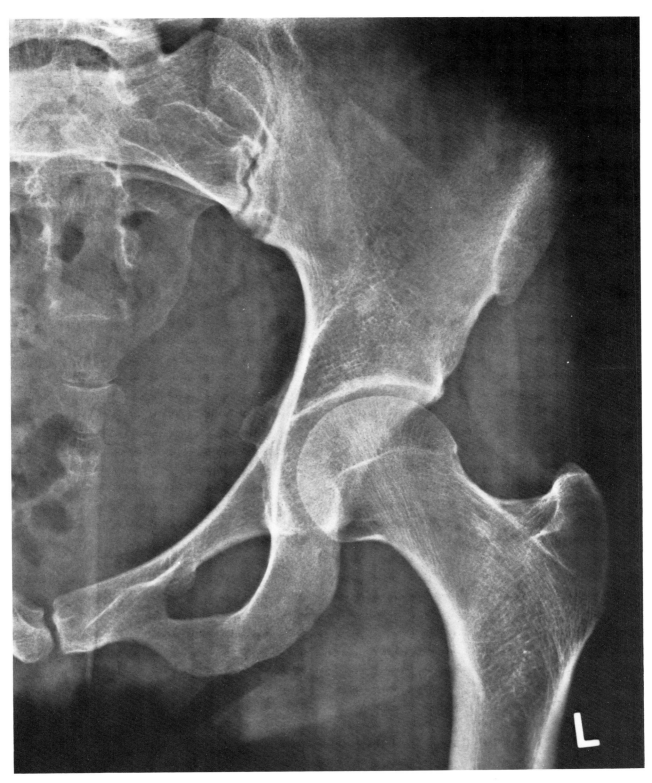

Fig. 84. Hip joint, a.p. view

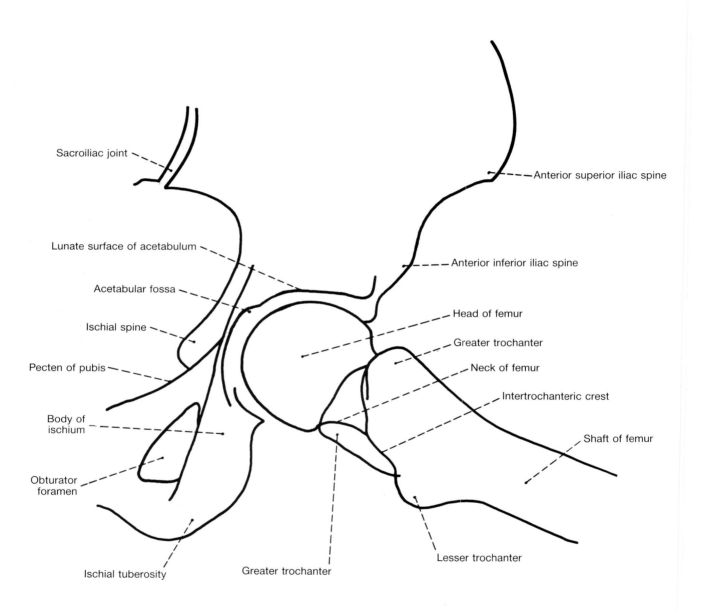

Sacroiliac joint

Anterior superior iliac spine

Lunate surface of acetabulum

Anterior inferior iliac spine

Acetabular fossa

Head of femur

Ischial spine

Greater trochanter

Pecten of pubis

Neck of femur

Intertrochanteric crest

Body of ischium

Shaft of femur

Obturator foramen

Ischial tuberosity

Greater trochanter

Lesser trochanter

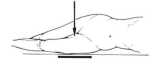

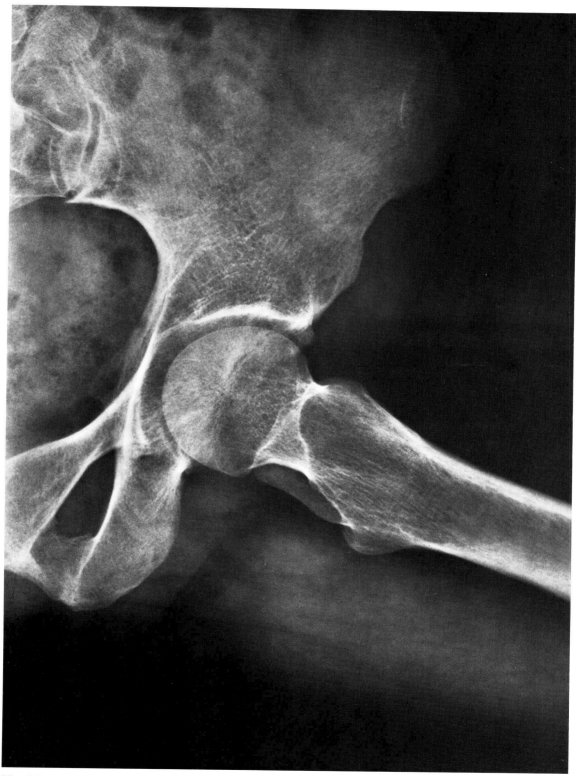

Fig. 85. Left hip joint with leg abducted laterally (Lauenstein or frog leg)

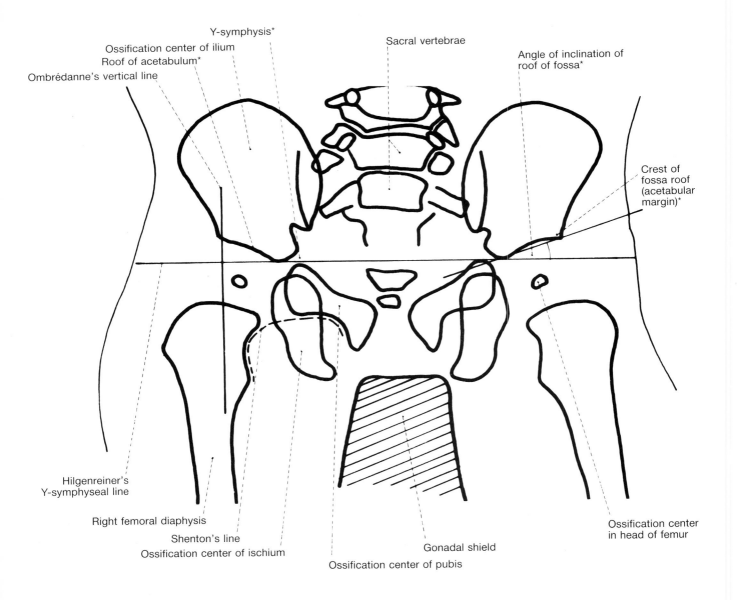

Y-symphysis*

Ossification center of ilium
Roof of acetabulum*

Ombrédanne's vertical line

Sacral vertebrae

Angle of inclination of
roof of fossa*

Crest of
fossa roof
(acetabular
margin)*

Hilgenreiner's
Y-symphyseal line

Right femoral diaphysis

Shenton's line
Ossification center of ischium

Gonadal shield

Ossification center of pubis

Ossification center
in head of femur

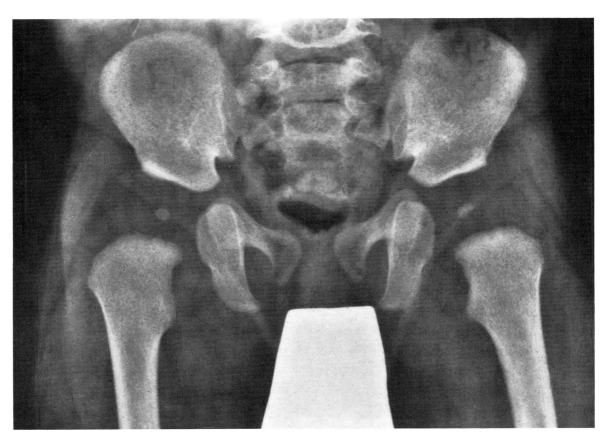

Fig. 86. Child's hip joint

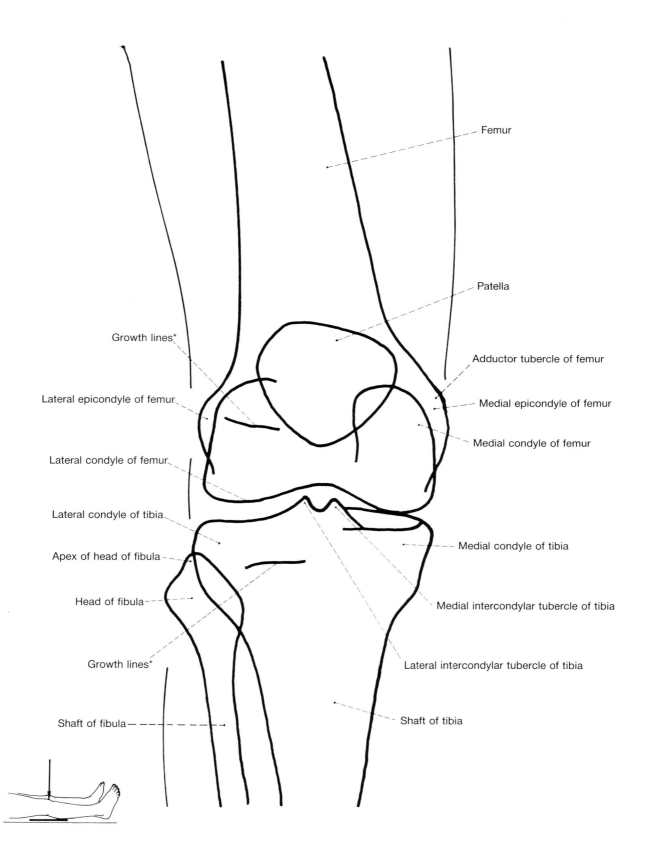

Femur

Patella

Growth lines*

Adductor tubercle of femur

Lateral epicondyle of femur

Medial epicondyle of femur

Medial condyle of femur

Lateral condyle of femur

Lateral condyle of tibia

Medial condyle of tibia

Apex of head of fibula

Head of fibula

Medial intercondylar tubercle of tibia

Lateral intercondylar tubercle of tibia

Growth lines*

Shaft of fibula

Shaft of tibia

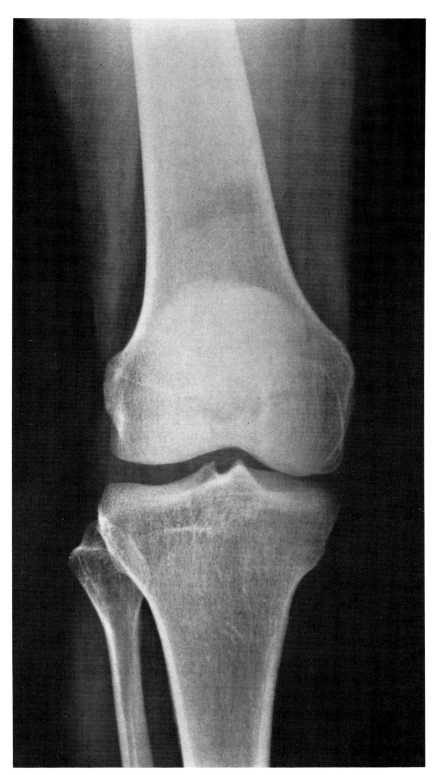

Fig. 87. Right knee joint, a.p. view

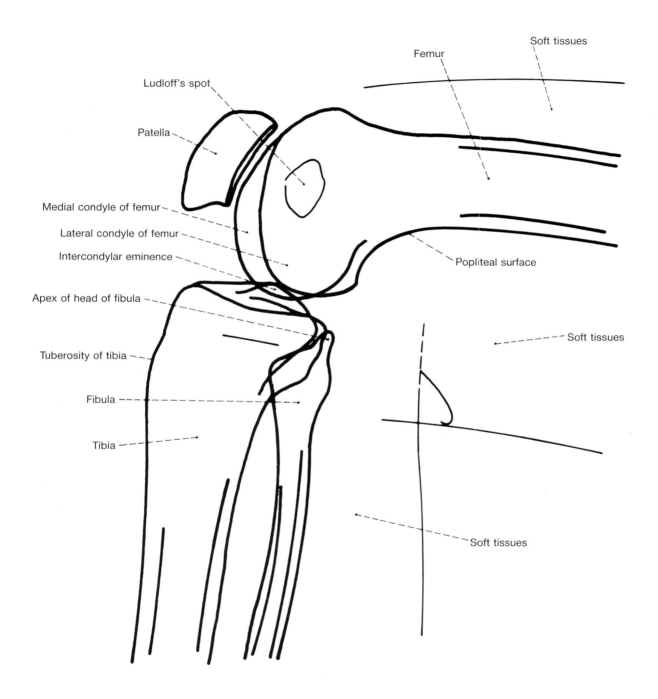

Soft tissues

Femur

Ludloff's spot

Patella

Medial condyle of femur

Lateral condyle of femur

Intercondylar eminence

Apex of head of fibula

Tuberosity of tibia

Fibula

Tibia

Popliteal surface

Soft tissues

Soft tissues

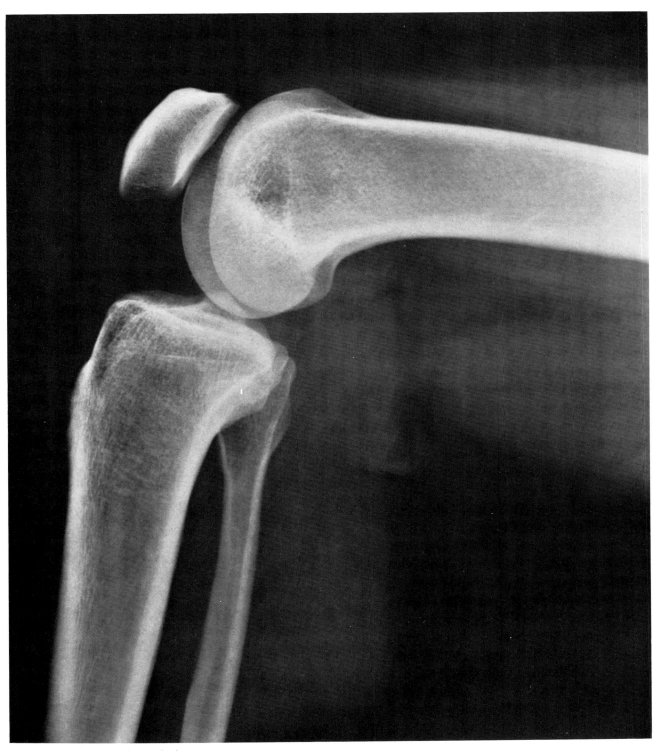

Fig. 88. Knee joint, lateral view

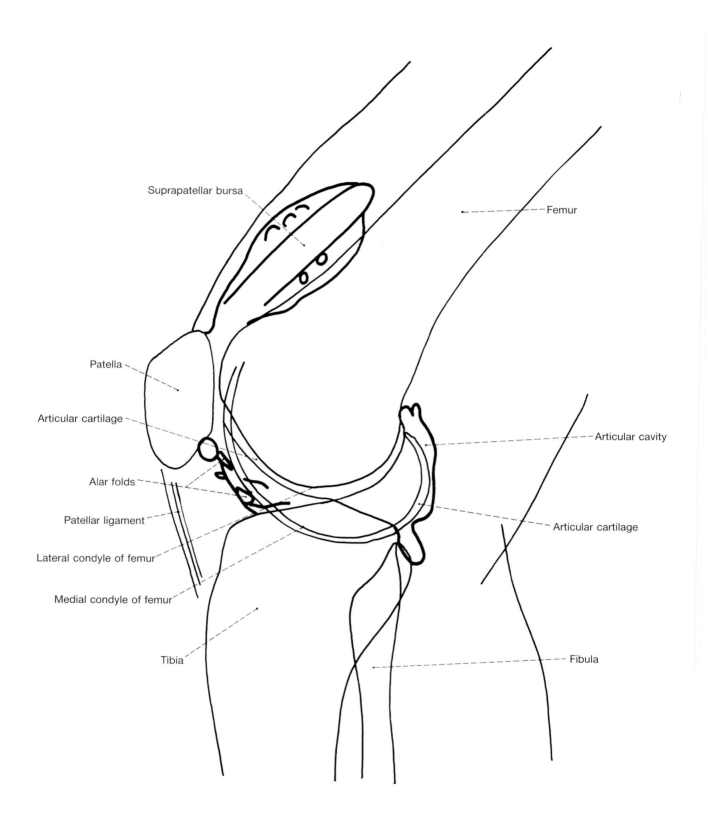

Suprapatellar bursa

Femur

Patella

Articular cartilage

Articular cavity

Alar folds

Patellar ligament

Articular cartilage

Lateral condyle of femur

Medial condyle of femur

Tibia

Fibula

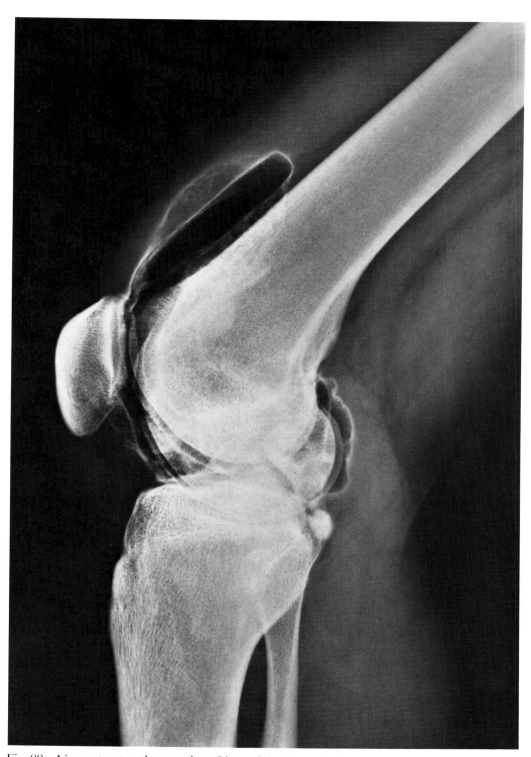

Fig. 89. Air contrast arthrography of knee joint, lateral view

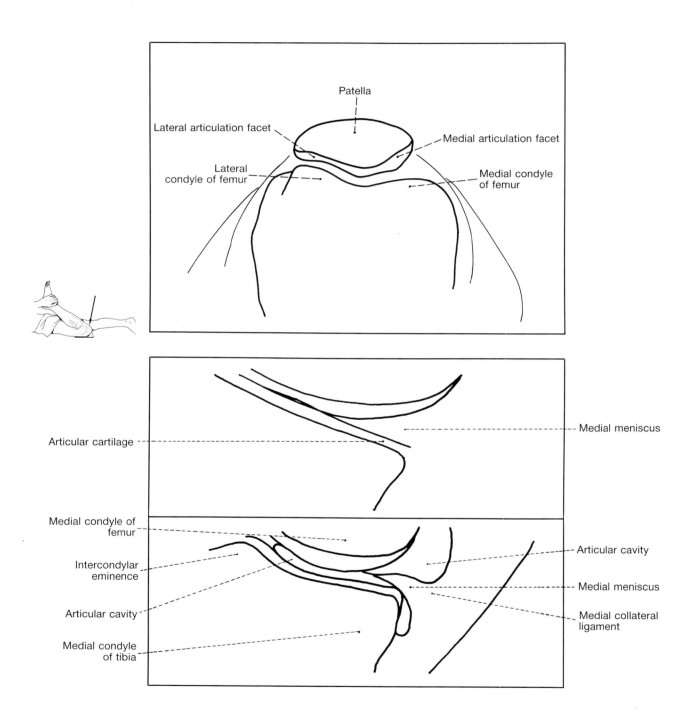

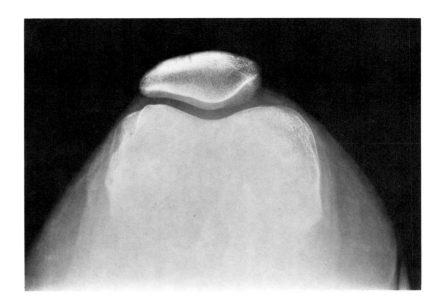

Fig. 90. Patella, axial view

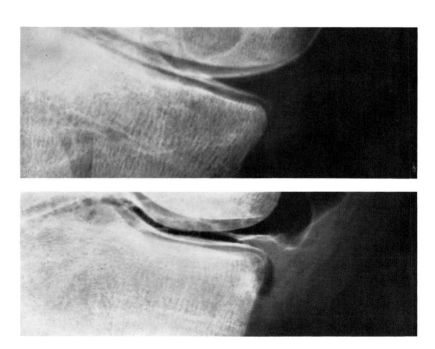

Fig. 91. Air contrast arthrography
of knee joint, a.p. view (coned-down
image of the medial meniscus)

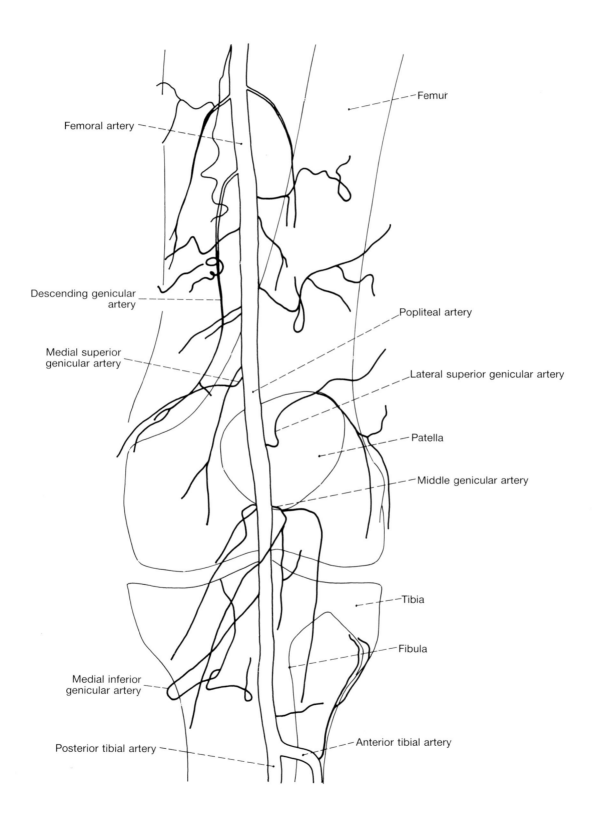

Femoral artery

Descending genicular artery

Medial superior genicular artery

Femur

Popliteal artery

Lateral superior genicular artery

Patella

Middle genicular artery

Tibia

Fibula

Medial inferior genicular artery

Posterior tibial artery

Anterior tibial artery

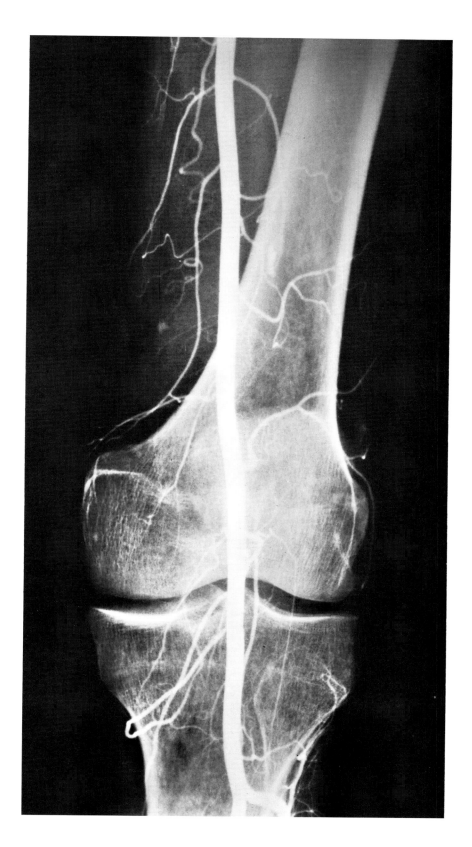

Fig. 92. Angiogram of left
knee joint, a.p. view

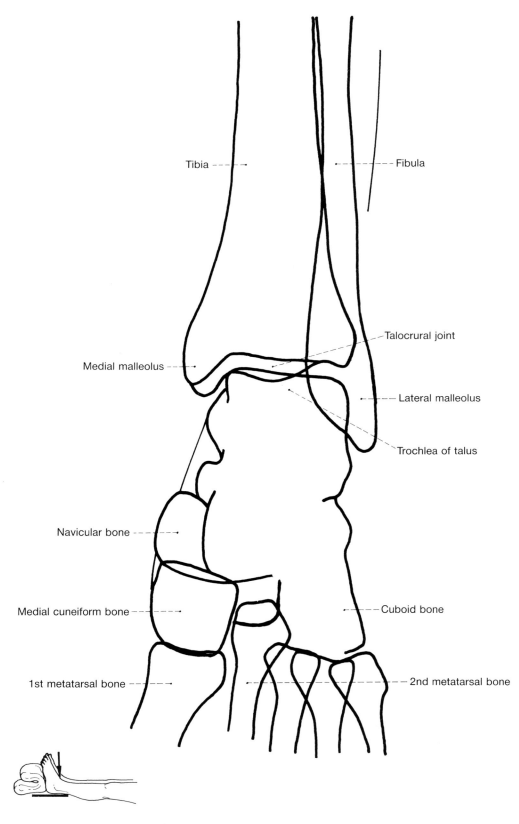

Tibia

Fibula

Talocrural joint

Medial malleolus

Lateral malleolus

Trochlea of talus

Navicular bone

Medial cuneiform bone

Cuboid bone

1st metatarsal bone

2nd metatarsal bone

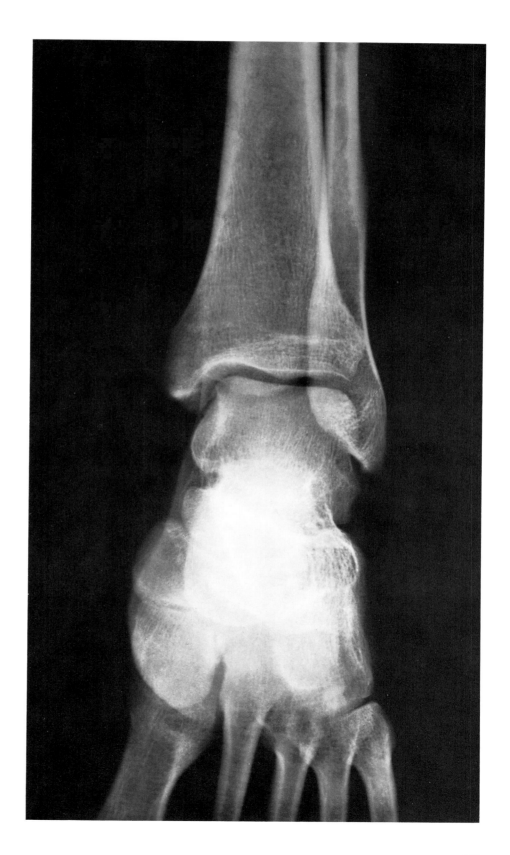

Fig. 93. Left ankle joint,
a.p. view

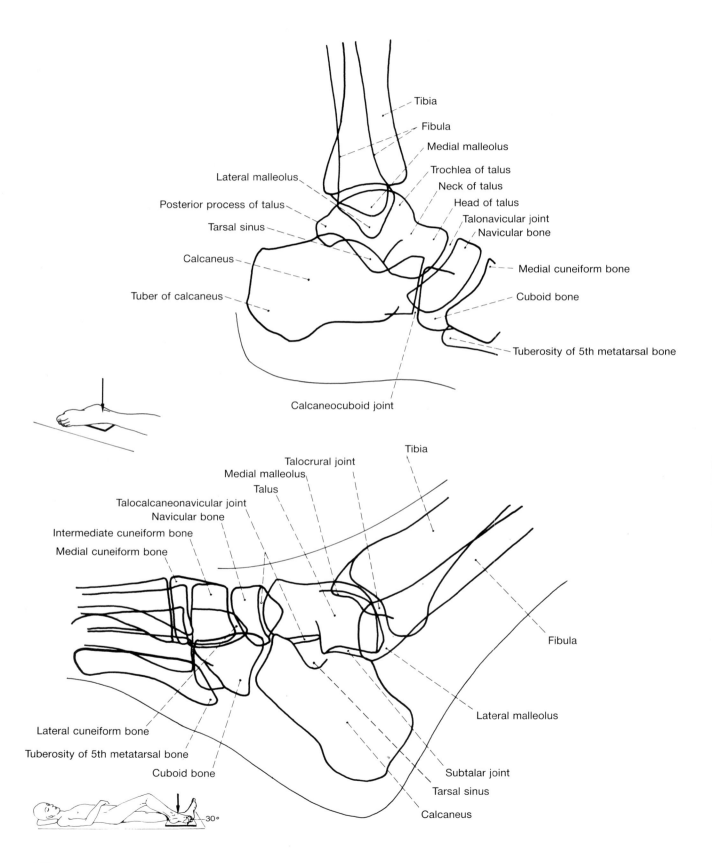

Tibia

Fibula

Medial malleolus

Trochlea of talus

Lateral malleolus

Neck of talus

Posterior process of talus

Head of talus

Talonavicular joint

Tarsal sinus

Navicular bone

Calcaneus

Medial cuneiform bone

Tuber of calcaneus

Cuboid bone

Tuberosity of 5th metatarsal bone

Calcaneocuboid joint

Tibia

Talocrural joint

Medial malleolus

Talus

Talocalcaneonavicular joint

Navicular bone

Intermediate cuneiform bone

Medial cuneiform bone

Fibula

Lateral malleolus

Lateral cuneiform bone

Tuberosity of 5th metatarsal bone

Subtalar joint

Cuboid bone

Tarsal sinus

Calcaneus

30°

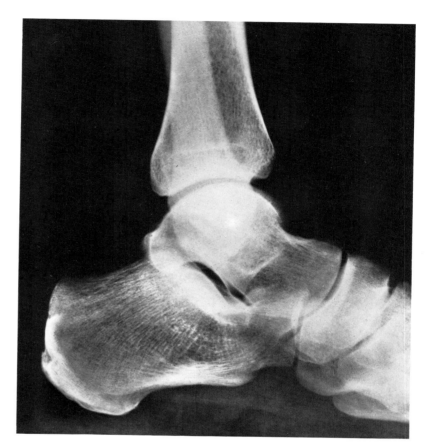

Fig. 94. Left ankle,
lateral view

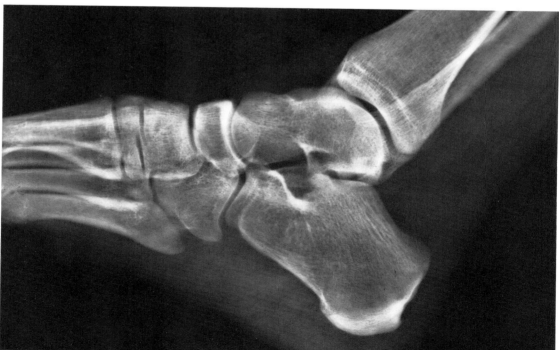

Fig. 95.
Right ankle
joint or tarsus,
oblique view

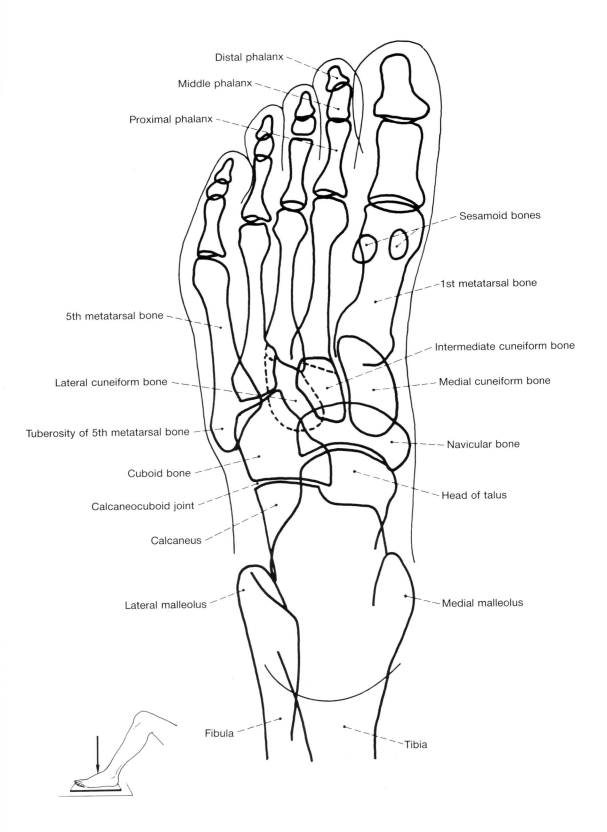

Distal phalanx

Middle phalanx

Proximal phalanx

Sesamoid bones

1st metatarsal bone

5th metatarsal bone

Intermediate cuneiform bone

Lateral cuneiform bone

Medial cuneiform bone

Tuberosity of 5th metatarsal bone

Navicular bone

Cuboid bone

Calcaneocuboid joint

Head of talus

Calcaneus

Lateral malleolus

Medial malleolus

Fibula

Tibia

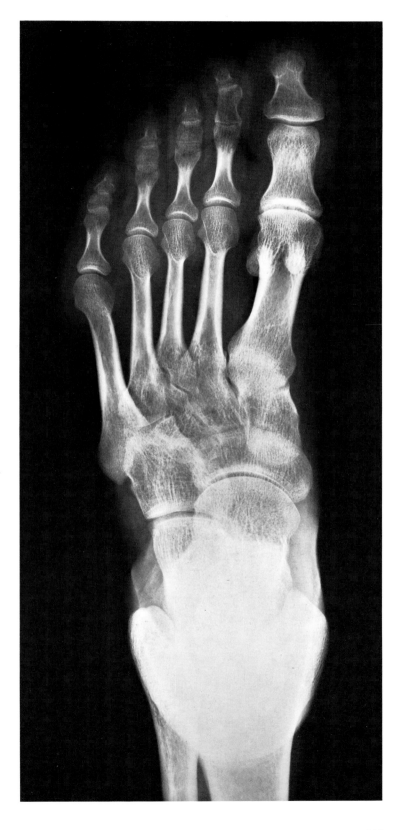

Fig. 96. Left foot, dorsoplantar view

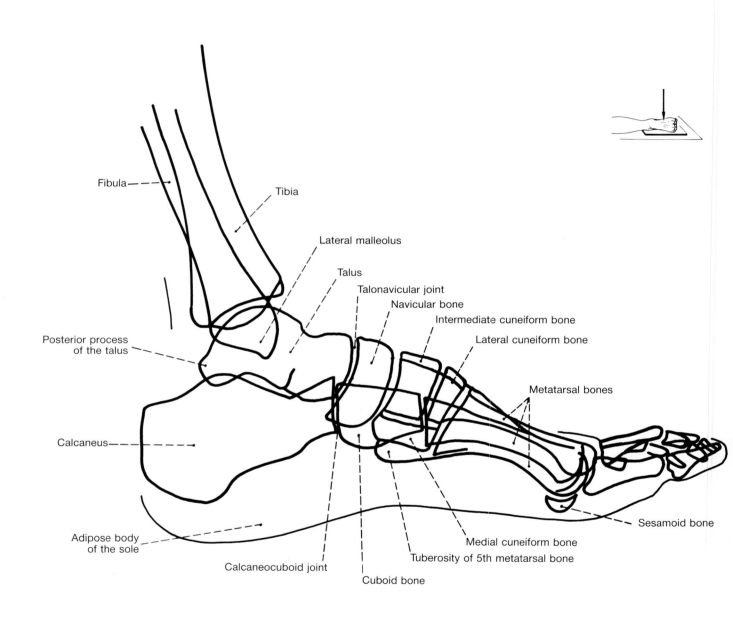

Fibula

Tibia

Lateral malleolus

Talus

Talonavicular joint

Navicular bone

Intermediate cuneiform bone

Lateral cuneiform bone

Posterior process
of the talus

Metatarsal bones

Calcaneus

Sesamoid bone

Adipose body
of the sole

Medial cuneiform bone

Calcaneocuboid joint

Tuberosity of 5th metatarsal bone

Cuboid bone

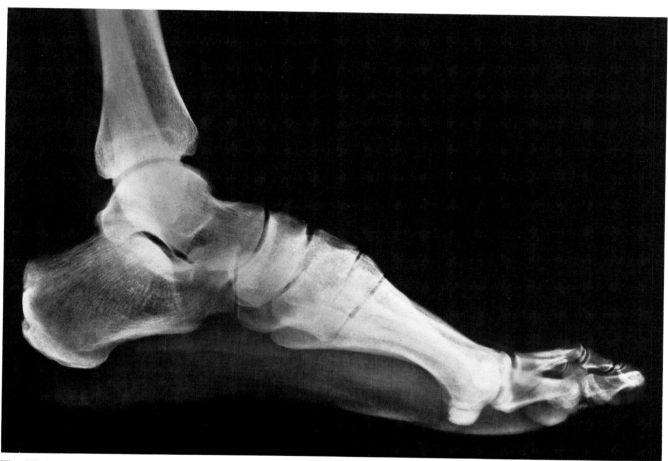

Fig. 97. Left foot, lateral view

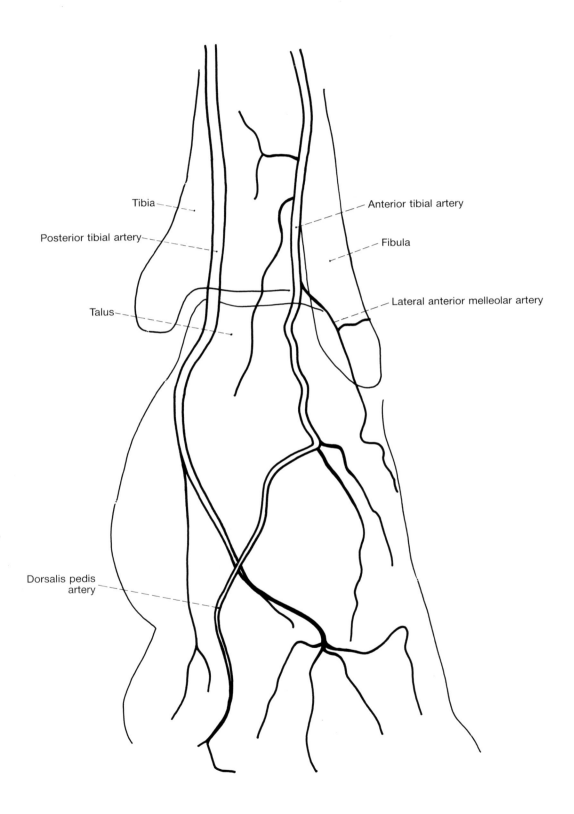

Tibia

Posterior tibial artery

Talus

Anterior tibial artery

Fibula

Lateral anterior melleolar artery

Dorsalis pedis
artery

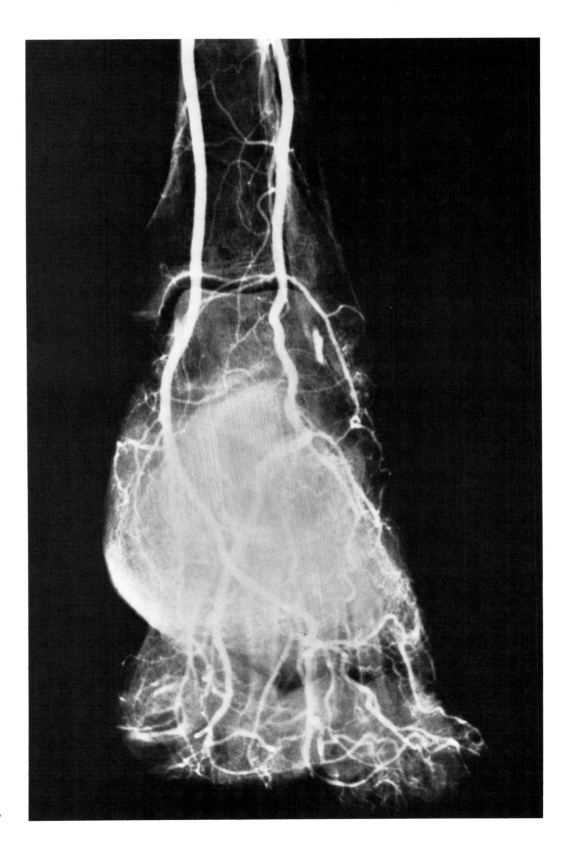

Fig. 98.
Angiogram of left
ankle joint, a.p. view

Thorax

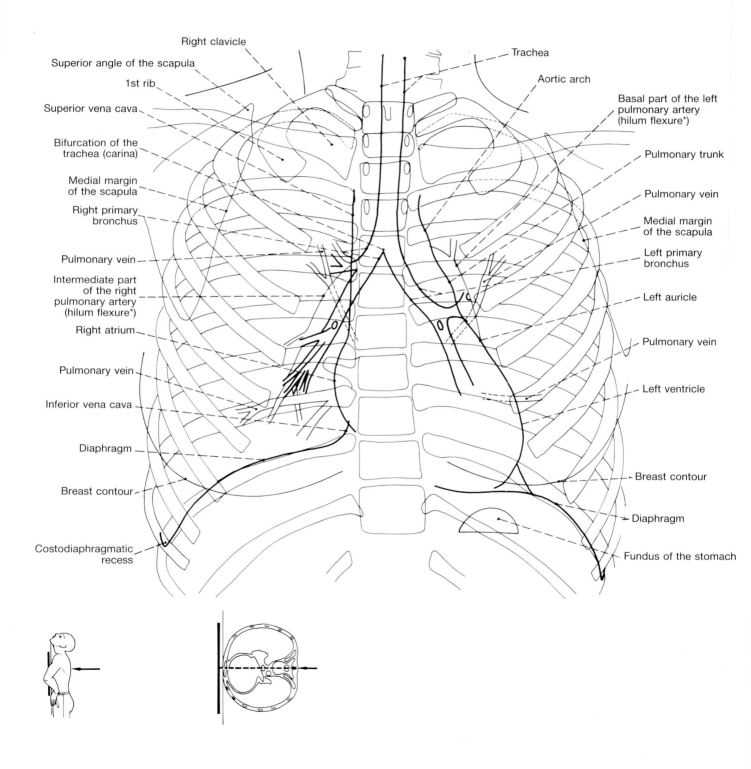

Right clavicle

Superior angle of the scapula

1st rib

Superior vena cava

Bifurcation of the trachea (carina)

Medial margin of the scapula

Right primary bronchus

Pulmonary vein

Intermediate part of the right pulmonary artery (hilum flexure*)

Right atrium

Pulmonary vein

Inferior vena cava

Diaphragm

Breast contour

Costodiaphragmatic recess

Trachea

Aortic arch

Basal part of the left pulmonary artery (hilum flexure*)

Pulmonary trunk

Pulmonary vein

Medial margin of the scapula

Left primary bronchus

Left auricle

Pulmonary vein

Left ventricle

Breast contour

Diaphragm

Fundus of the stomach

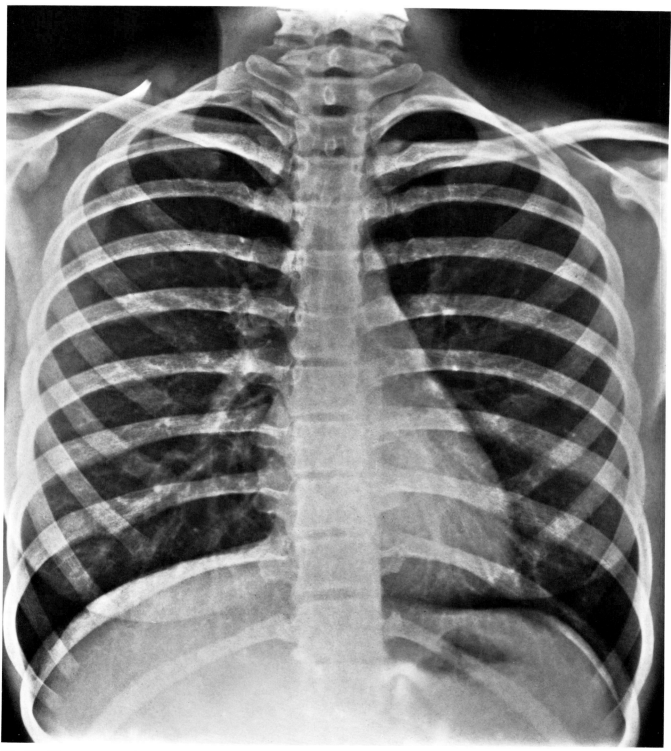

Fig. 99. Thorax, p.a. view

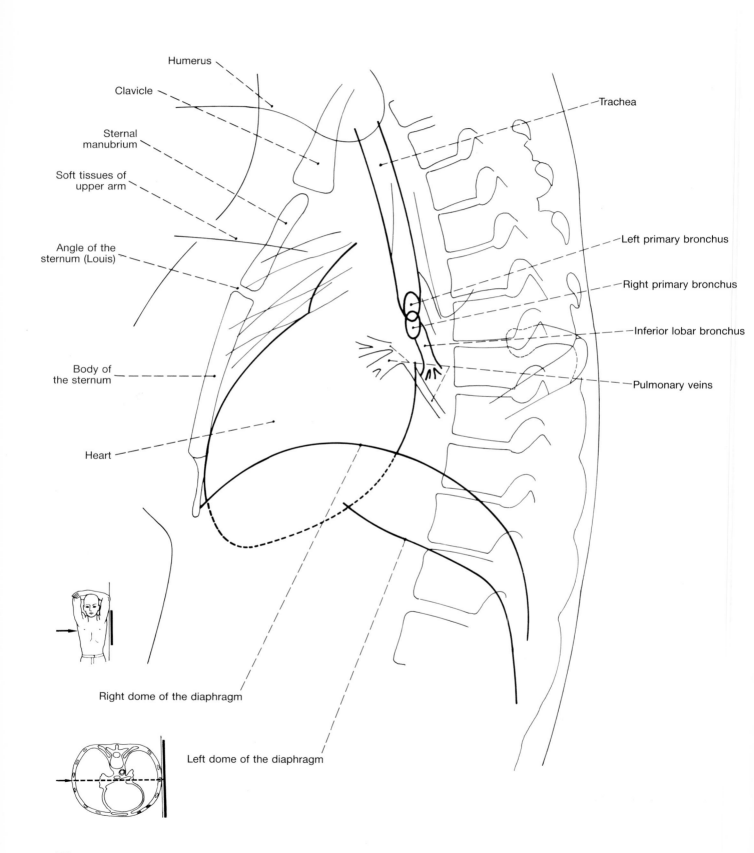

Humerus

Clavicle

Sternal manubrium

Soft tissues of upper arm

Angle of the sternum (Louis)

Body of the sternum

Heart

Trachea

Left primary bronchus

Right primary bronchus

Inferior lobar bronchus

Pulmonary veins

Right dome of the diaphragm

Left dome of the diaphragm

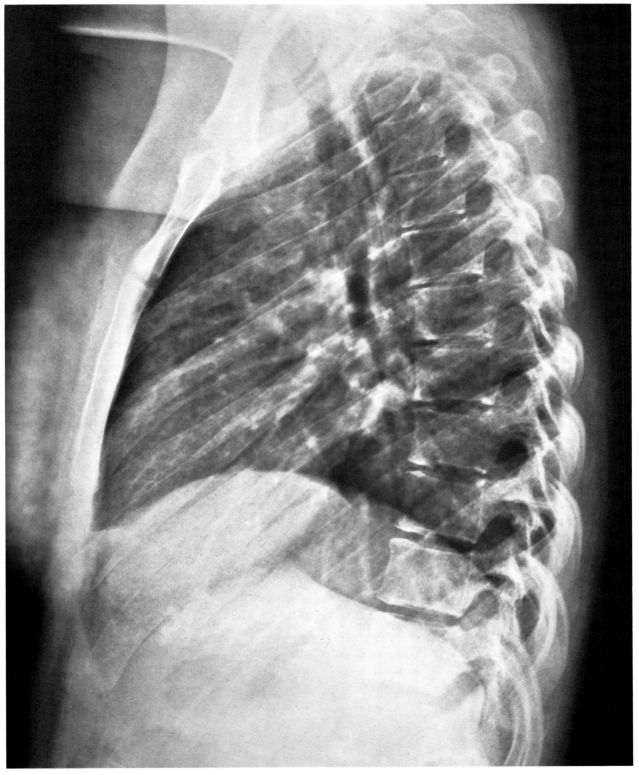

Fig. 100. Thorax, lateral view

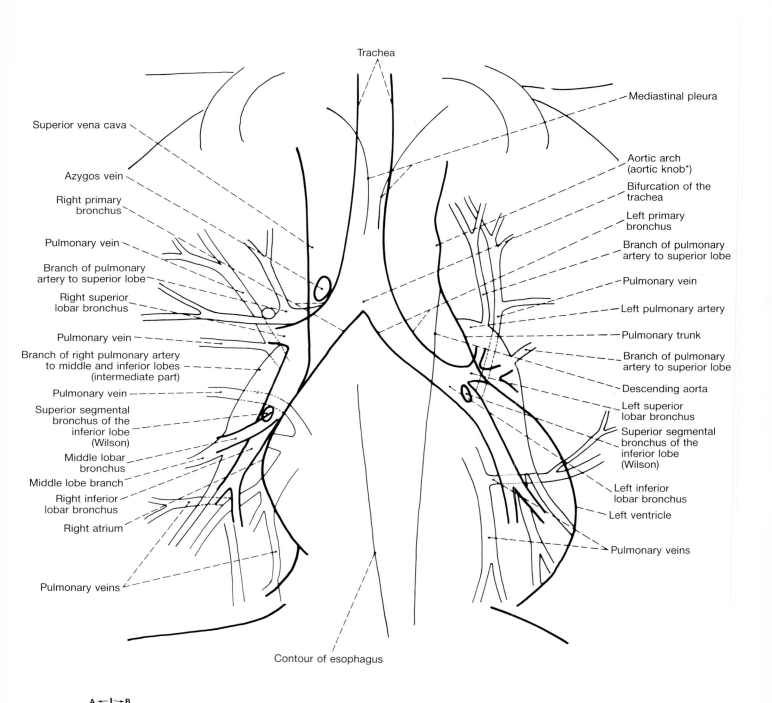

Trachea

Mediastinal pleura

Superior vena cava

Aortic arch
(aortic knob*)

Azygos vein

Bifurcation of the
trachea

Right primary
bronchus

Left primary
bronchus

Pulmonary vein

Branch of pulmonary
artery to superior lobe

Branch of pulmonary
artery to superior lobe

Pulmonary vein

Right superior
lobar bronchus

Left pulmonary artery

Pulmonary vein

Pulmonary trunk

Branch of right pulmonary artery
to middle and inferior lobes
(intermediate part)

Branch of pulmonary
artery to superior lobe

Pulmonary vein

Descending aorta

Superior segmental
bronchus of the
inferior lobe
(Wilson)

Left superior
lobar bronchus

Superior segmental
bronchus of the
inferior lobe
(Wilson)

Middle lobar
bronchus

Middle lobe branch

Left inferior
lobar bronchus

Right inferior
lobar bronchus

Left ventricle

Right atrium

Pulmonary veins

Pulmonary veins

Contour of esophagus

A ←|→ B

B ←   → A

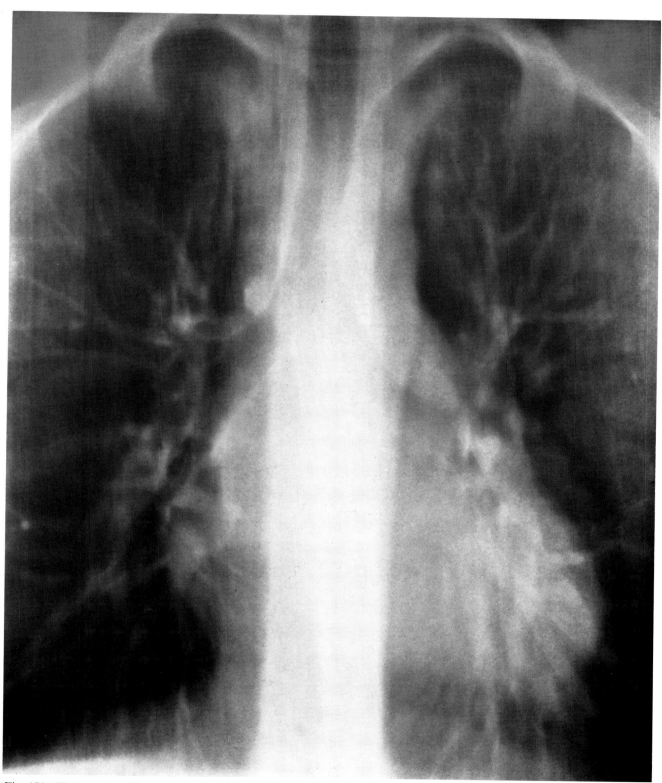

Fig. 101. Tomogram of lungs, a.p. view

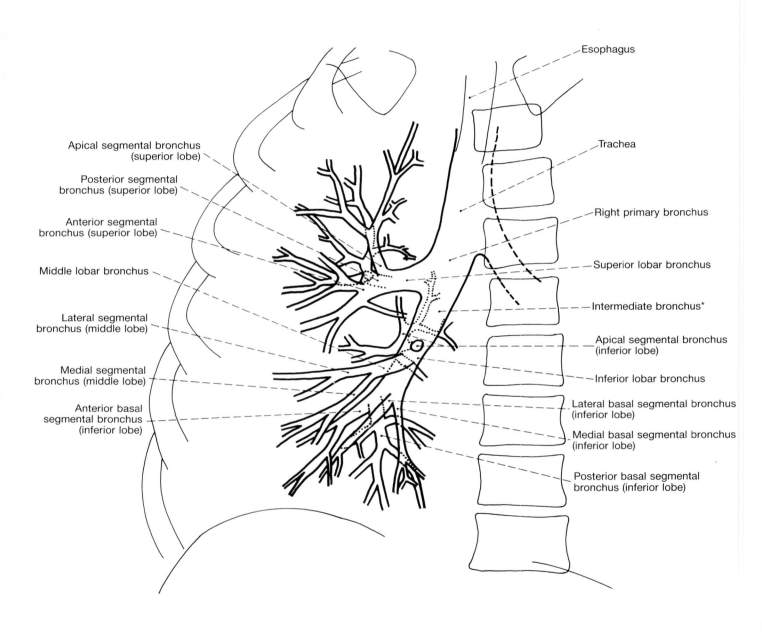

Esophagus

Trachea

Right primary bronchus

Superior lobar bronchus

Intermediate bronchus*

Apical segmental bronchus
(inferior lobe)

Inferior lobar bronchus

Lateral basal segmental bronchus
(inferior lobe)

Medial basal segmental bronchus
(inferior lobe)

Posterior basal segmental
bronchus (inferior lobe)

Apical segmental bronchus
(superior lobe)

Posterior segmental
bronchus (superior lobe)

Anterior segmental
bronchus (superior lobe)

Middle lobar bronchus

Lateral segmental
bronchus (middle lobe)

Medial segmental
bronchus (middle lobe)

Anterior basal
segmental bronchus
(inferior lobe)

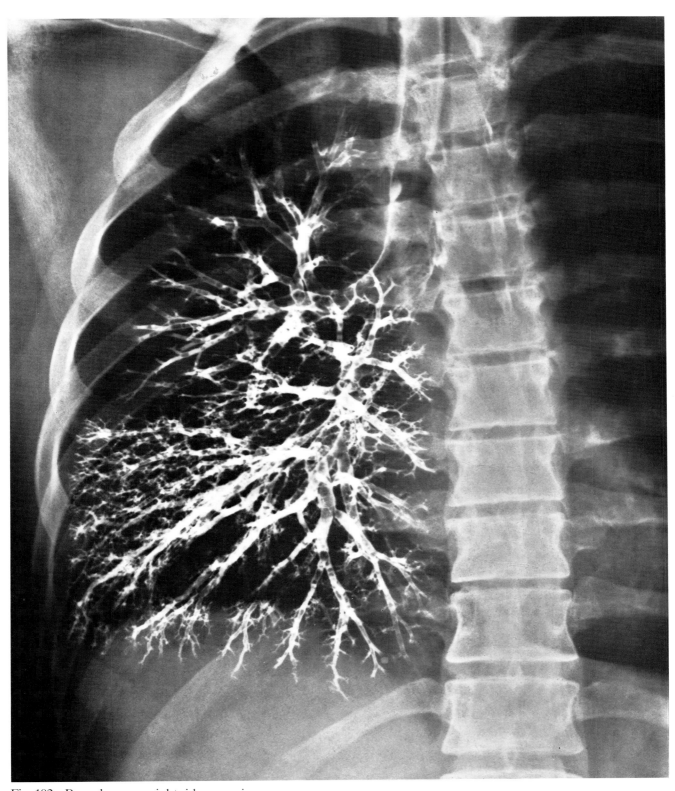

Fig. 102. Bronchogram, right side, a.p. view

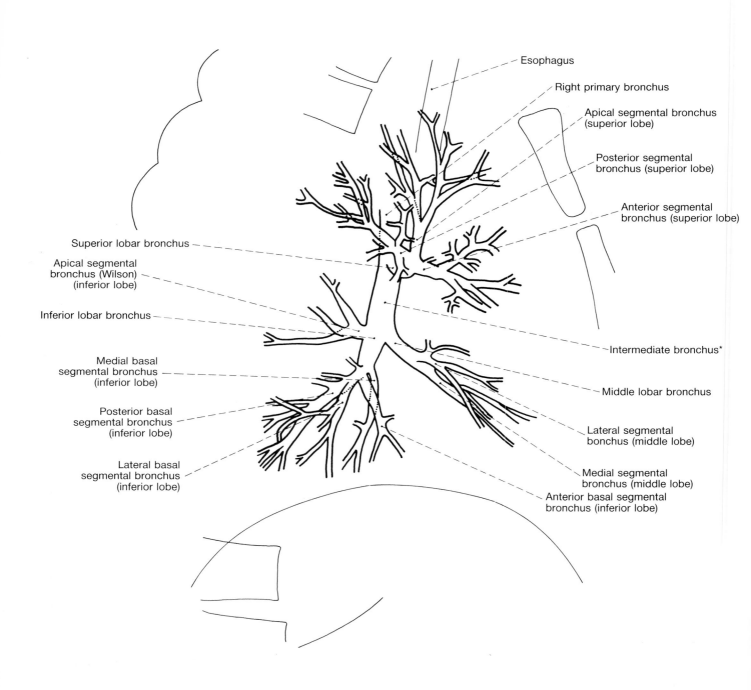

Esophagus

Right primary bronchus

Apical segmental bronchus
(superior lobe)

Posterior segmental
bronchus (superior lobe)

Anterior segmental
bronchus (superior lobe)

Superior lobar bronchus

Apical segmental
bronchus (Wilson)
(inferior lobe)

Inferior lobar bronchus

Intermediate bronchus*

Medial basal
segmental bronchus
(inferior lobe)

Middle lobar bronchus

Posterior basal
segmental bronchus
(inferior lobe)

Lateral segmental
bonchus (middle lobe)

Lateral basal
segmental bronchus
(inferior lobe)

Medial segmental
bronchus (middle lobe)

Anterior basal segmental
bronchus (inferior lobe)

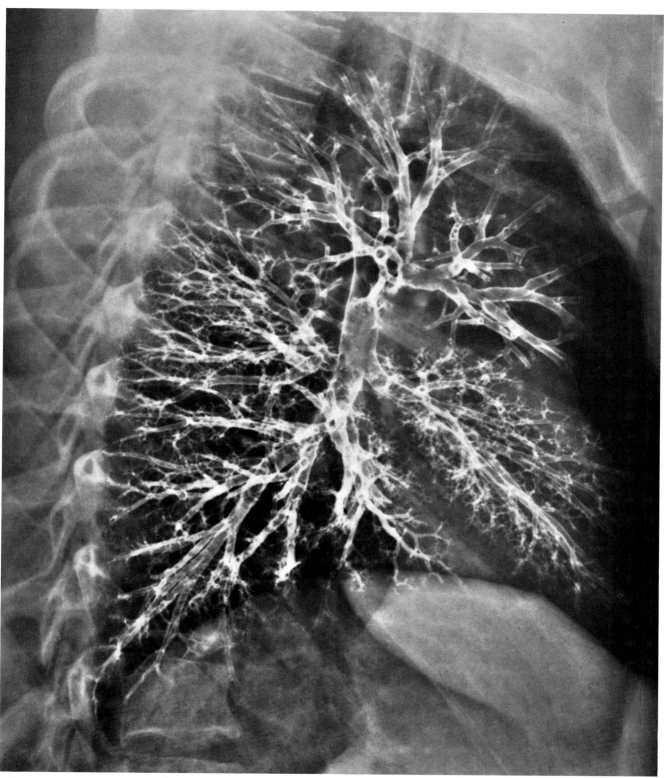

Fig. 103. Bronchogram, right side, slight oblique view

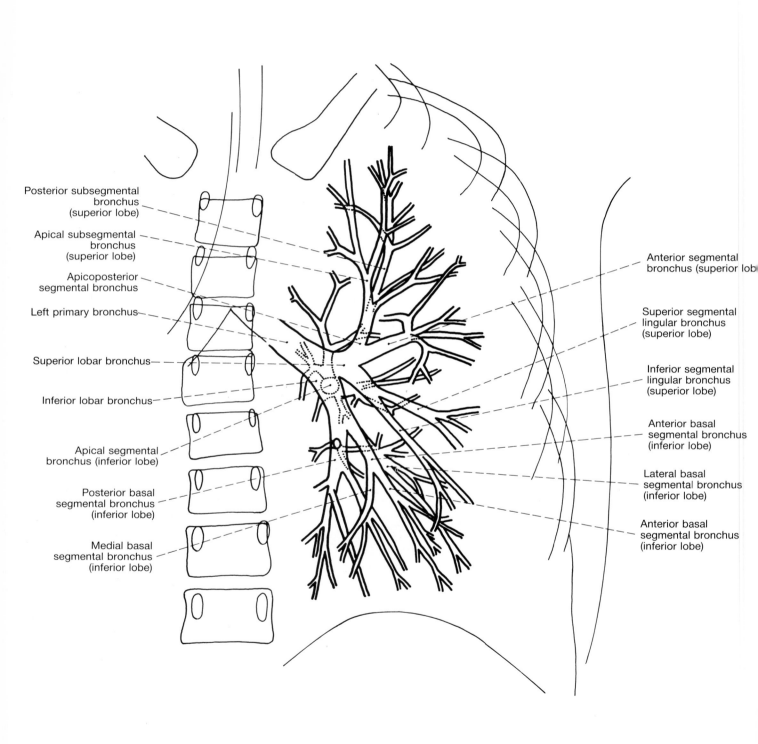

Posterior subsegmental
bronchus
(superior lobe)

Apical subsegmental
bronchus
(superior lobe)

Apicoposterior
segmental bronchus

Left primary bronchus

Superior lobar bronchus

Inferior lobar bronchus

Apical segmental
bronchus (inferior lobe)

Posterior basal
segmental bronchus
(inferior lobe)

Medial basal
segmental bronchus
(inferior lobe)

Anterior segmental
bronchus (superior lob

Superior segmental
lingular bronchus
(superior lobe)

Inferior segmental
lingular bronchus
(superior lobe)

Anterior basal
segmental bronchus
(inferior lobe)

Lateral basal
segmental bronchus
(inferior lobe)

Anterior basal
segmental bronchus
(inferior lobe)

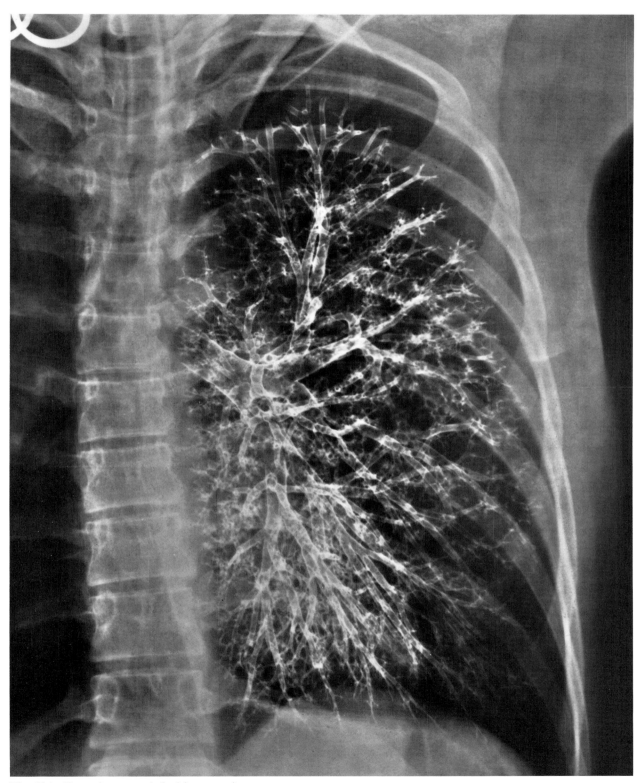

Fig. 104. Bronchogram, left side, a.p. view

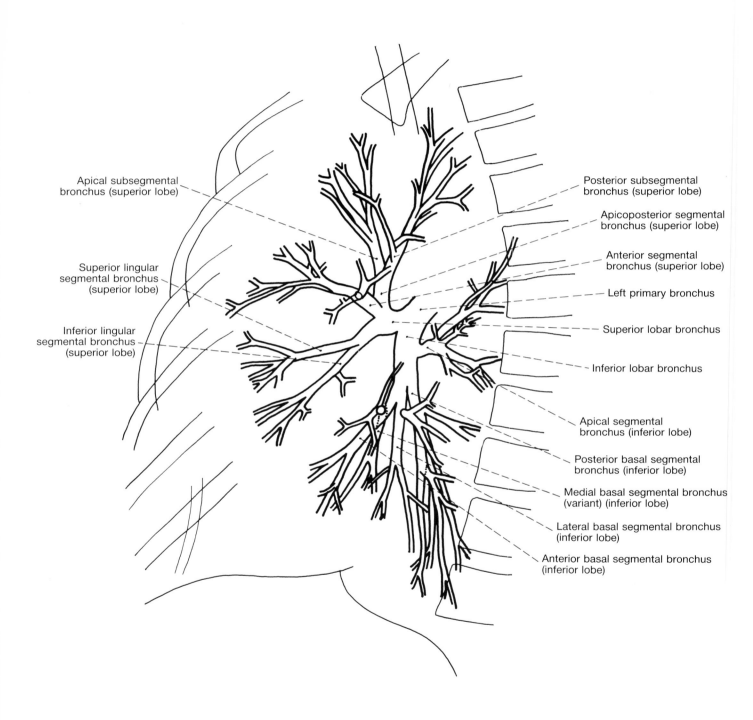

Apical subsegmental
bronchus (superior lobe)

Superior lingular
segmental bronchus
(superior lobe)

Inferior lingular
segmental bronchus
(superior lobe)

Posterior subsegmental
bronchus (superior lobe)

Apicoposterior segmental
bronchus (superior lobe)

Anterior segmental
bronchus (superior lobe)

Left primary bronchus

Superior lobar bronchus

Inferior lobar bronchus

Apical segmental
bronchus (inferior lobe)

Posterior basal segmental
bronchus (inferior lobe)

Medial basal segmental bronchus
(variant) (inferior lobe)

Lateral basal segmental bronchus
(inferior lobe)

Anterior basal segmental bronchus
(inferior lobe)

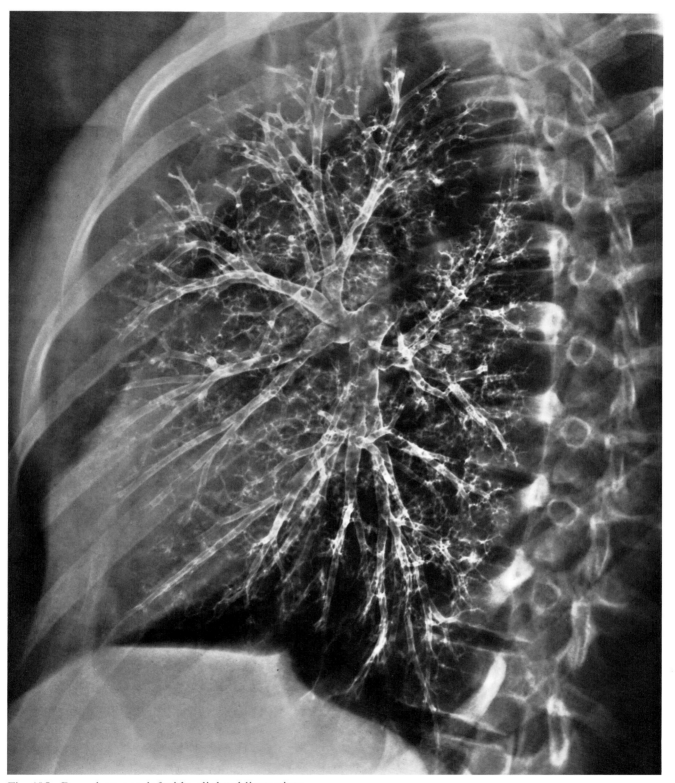

Fig. 105. Bronchogram, left side, slight oblique view

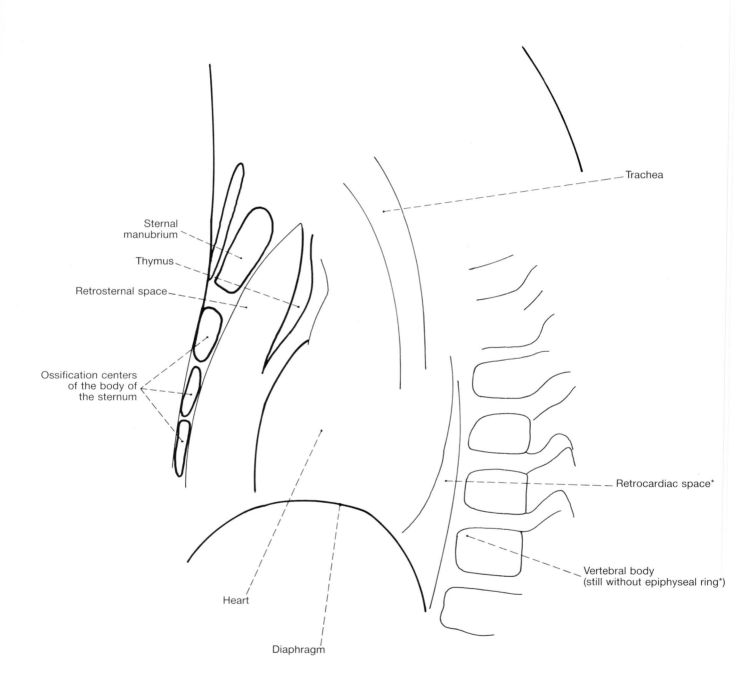

Sternal manubrium

Thymus

Retrosternal space

Ossification centers of the body of the sternum

Heart

Diaphragm

Trachea

Retrocardiac space*

Vertebral body (still without epiphyseal ring*)

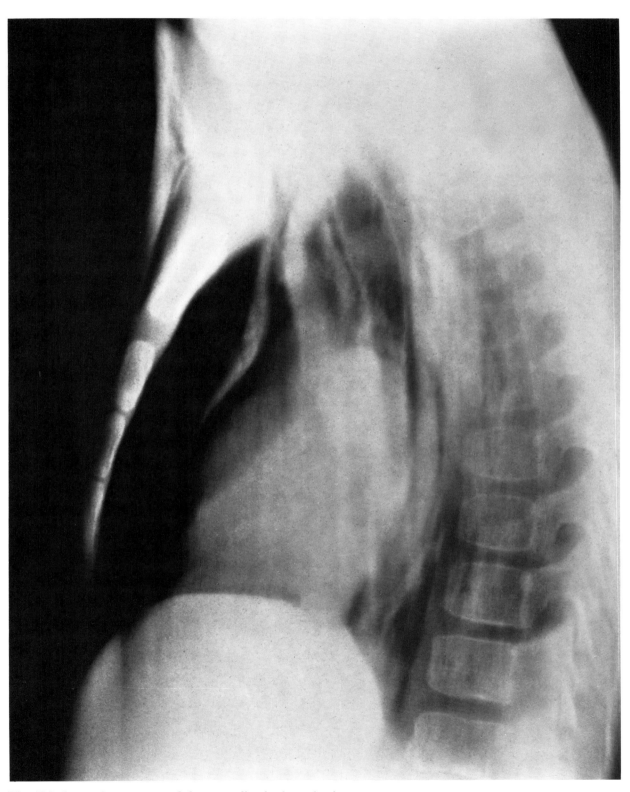

Fig. 106. Lateral tomogram of chest, mediastinal emphasis

Heart

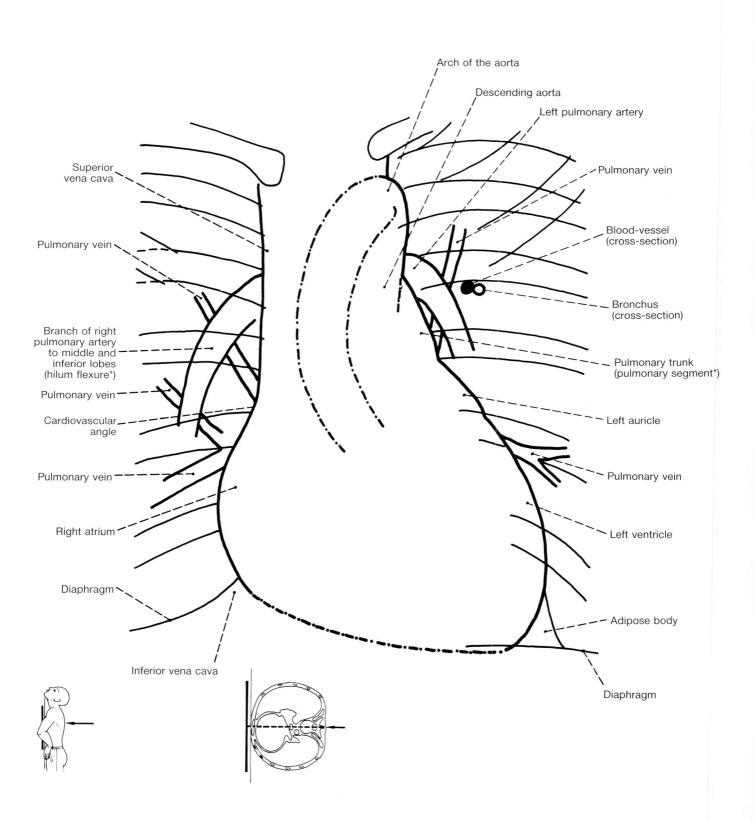

Arch of the aorta

Descending aorta

Left pulmonary artery

Superior vena cava

Pulmonary vein

Blood-vessel (cross-section)

Pulmonary vein

Bronchus (cross-section)

Branch of right pulmonary artery to middle and inferior lobes (hilum flexure*)

Pulmonary trunk (pulmonary segment*)

Pulmonary vein

Left auricle

Cardiovascular angle

Pulmonary vein

Pulmonary vein

Right atrium

Left ventricle

Diaphragm

Adipose body

Inferior vena cava

Diaphragm

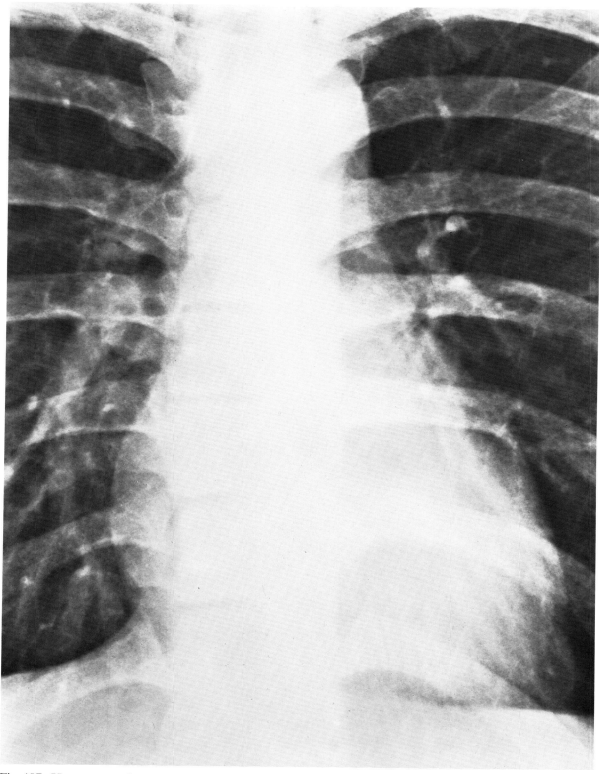

Fig. 107. Heart, p.a. view

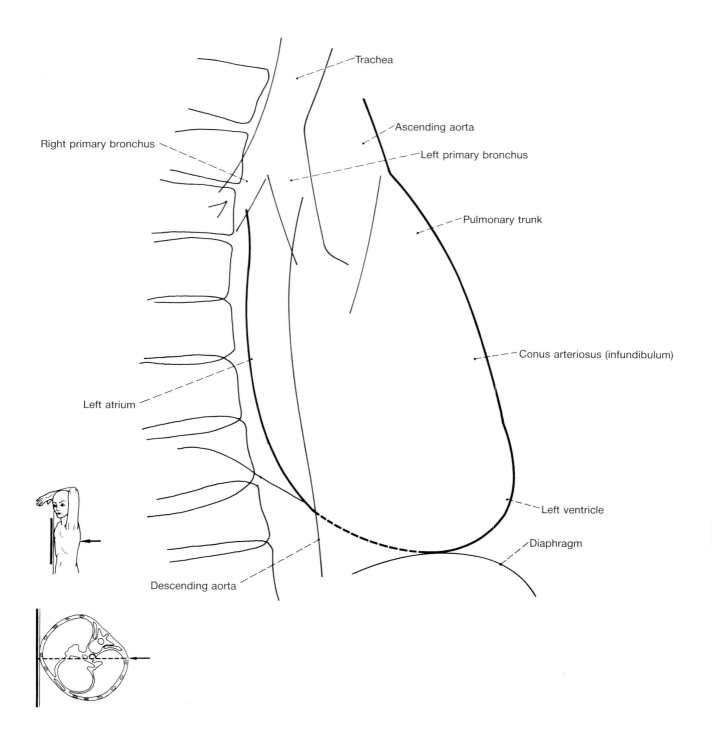

Trachea

Ascending aorta

Right primary bronchus

Left primary bronchus

Pulmonary trunk

Conus arteriosus (infundibulum)

Left atrium

Left ventricle

Diaphragm

Descending aorta

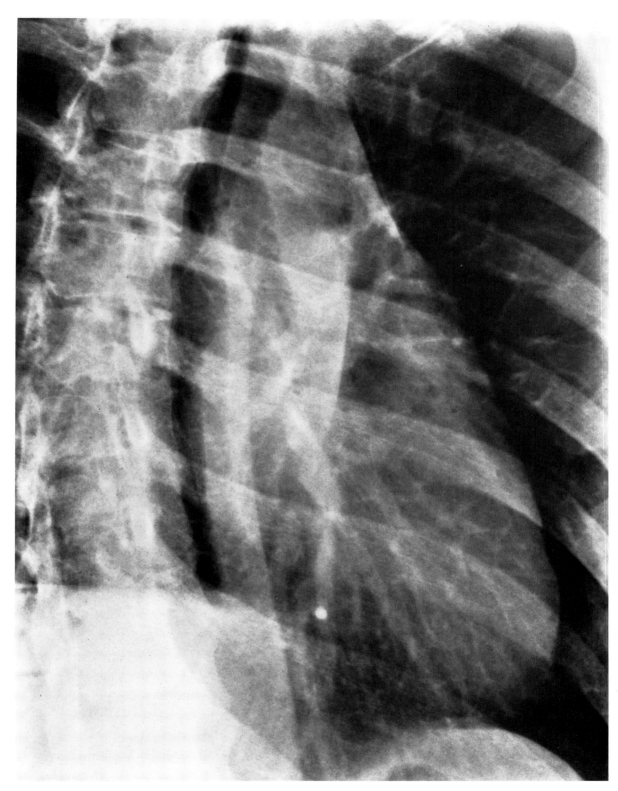

Fig. 108. Heart, right anterior oblique view

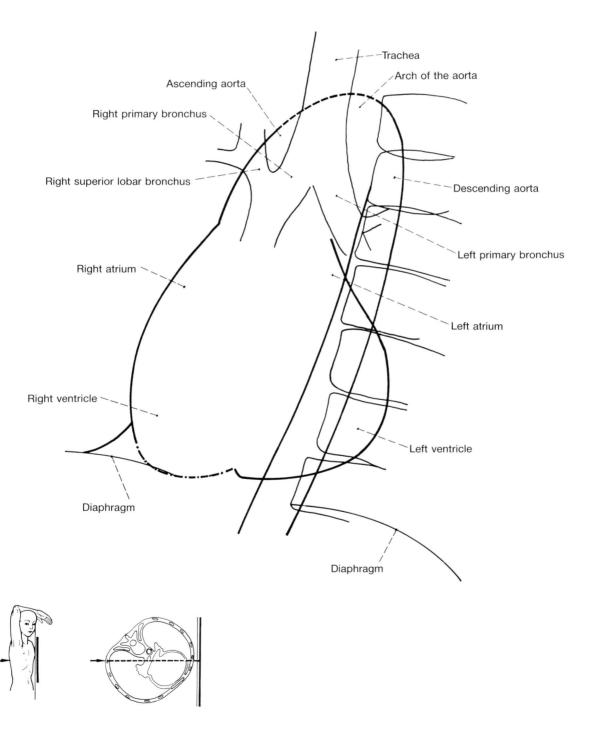

Trachea

Arch of the aorta

Ascending aorta

Right primary bronchus

Descending aorta

Right superior lobar bronchus

Left primary bronchus

Right atrium

Left atrium

Right ventricle

Left ventricle

Diaphragm

Diaphragm

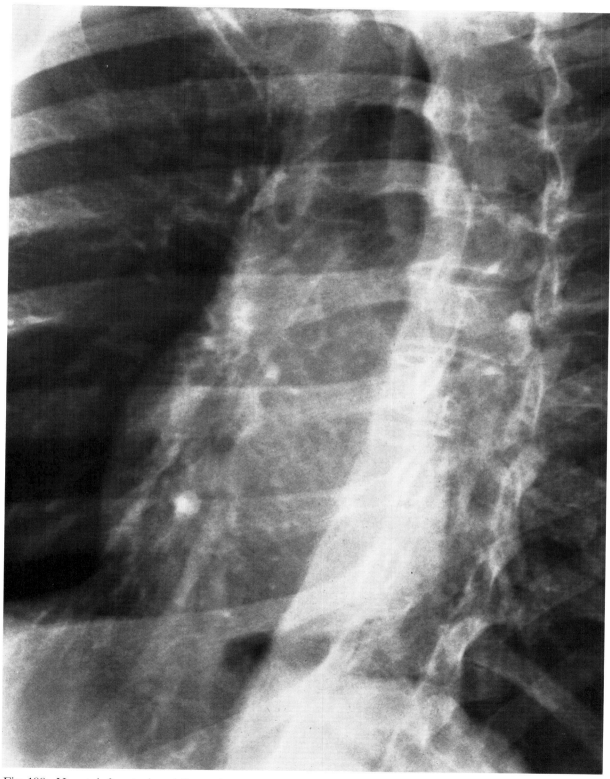

Fig. 109. Heart, left anterior oblique view

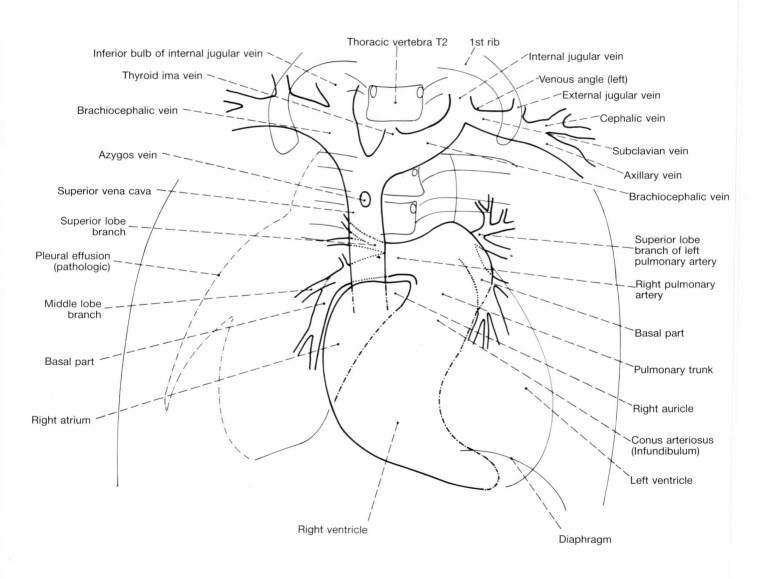

Inferior bulb of internal jugular vein

Thyroid ima vein

Brachiocephalic vein

Azygos vein

Superior vena cava

Superior lobe branch

Pleural effusion (pathologic)

Middle lobe branch

Basal part

Right atrium

Thoracic vertebra T2

1st rib

Internal jugular vein

Venous angle (left)

External jugular vein

Cephalic vein

Subclavian vein

Axillary vein

Brachiocephalic vein

Superior lobe branch of left pulmonary artery

Right pulmonary artery

Basal part

Pulmonary trunk

Right auricle

Conus arteriosus (Infundibulum)

Left ventricle

Right ventricle

Diaphragm

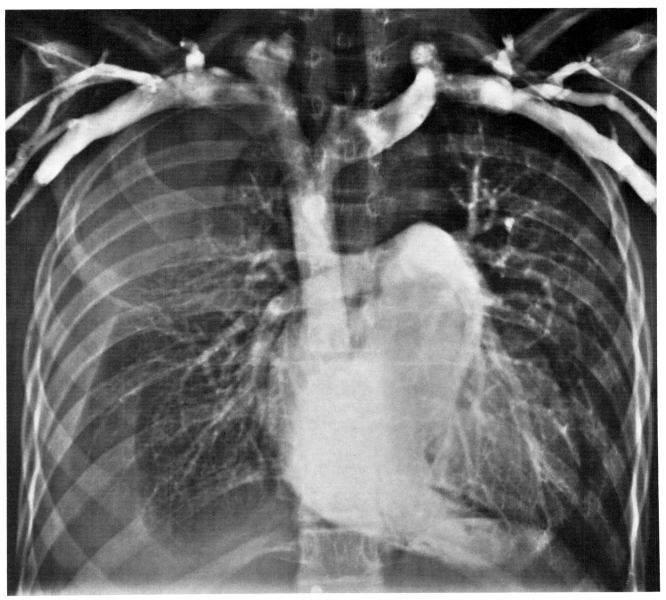

Fig. 110. Peripheral angiocardiogram of right ventricle

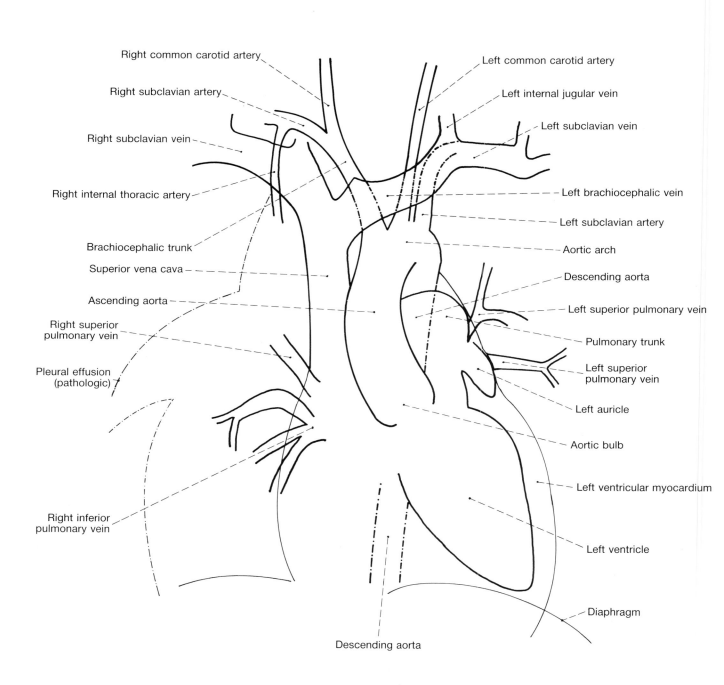

Right common carotid artery

Right subclavian artery

Right subclavian vein

Right internal thoracic artery

Brachiocephalic trunk

Superior vena cava

Ascending aorta

Right superior
pulmonary vein

Pleural effusion
(pathologic)

Right inferior
pulmonary vein

Left common carotid artery

Left internal jugular vein

Left subclavian vein

Left brachiocephalic vein

Left subclavian artery

Aortic arch

Descending aorta

Left superior pulmonary vein

Pulmonary trunk

Left superior
pulmonary vein

Left auricle

Aortic bulb

Left ventricular myocardium

Left ventricle

Diaphragm

Descending aorta

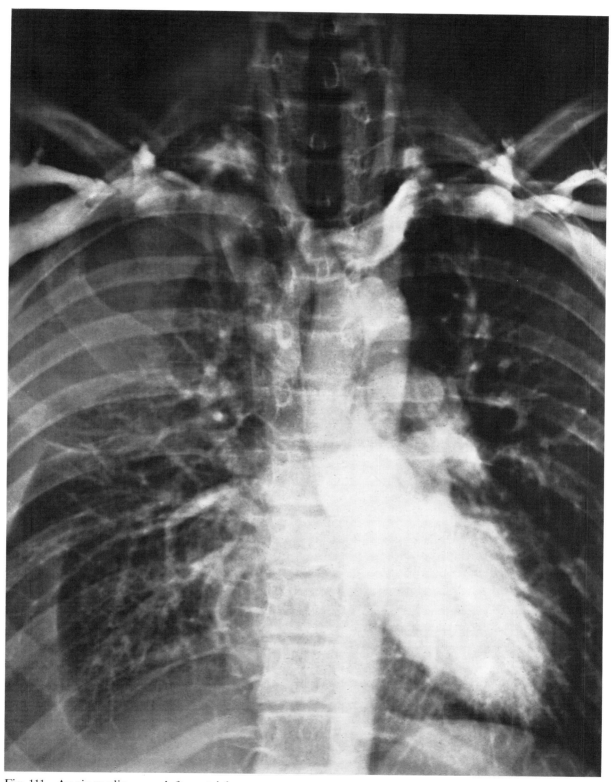

Fig. 111. Angiocardiogram, left ventricle

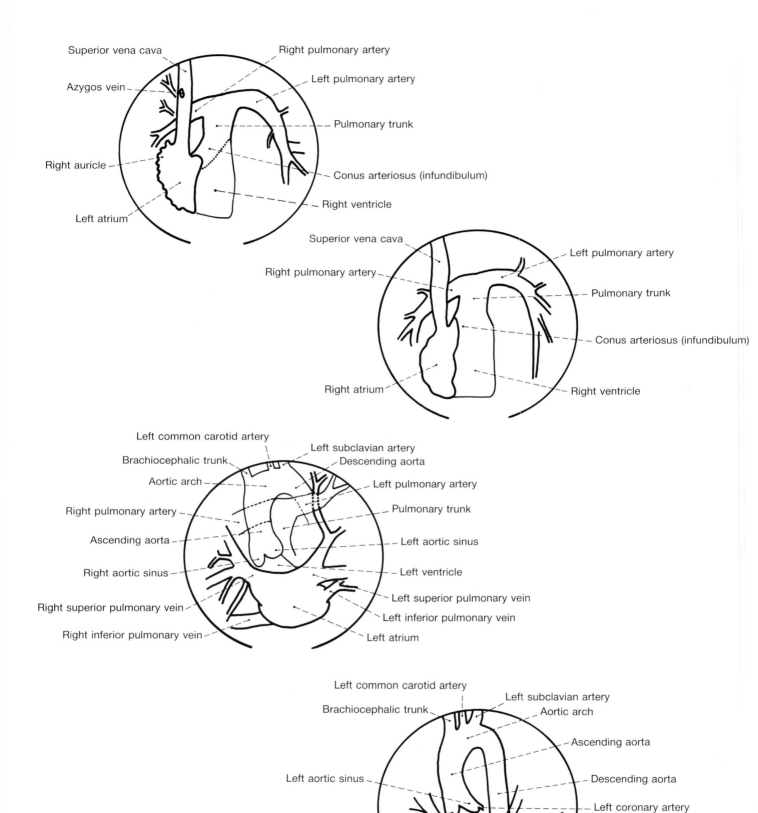

Superior vena cava

Azygos vein

Right pulmonary artery

Left pulmonary artery

Pulmonary trunk

Right auricle

Conus arteriosus (infundibulum)

Left atrium

Right ventricle

Superior vena cava

Right pulmonary artery

Left pulmonary artery

Pulmonary trunk

Conus arteriosus (infundibulum)

Right atrium

Right ventricle

Left common carotid artery

Brachiocephalic trunk

Left subclavian artery

Descending aorta

Aortic arch

Left pulmonary artery

Right pulmonary artery

Pulmonary trunk

Ascending aorta

Left aortic sinus

Right aortic sinus

Left ventricle

Right superior pulmonary vein

Left superior pulmonary vein

Right inferior pulmonary vein

Left inferior pulmonary vein

Left atrium

Left common carotid artery

Left subclavian artery

Brachiocephalic trunk

Aortic arch

Ascending aorta

Left aortic sinus

Descending aorta

Left coronary artery

Right aortic sinus

Left superior pulmonary vein

Right superior pulmonary vein

Left ventricle

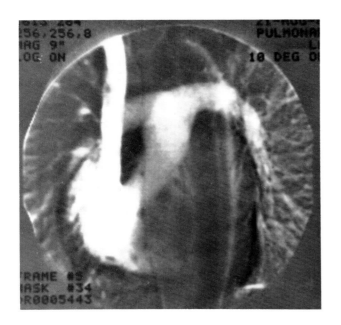
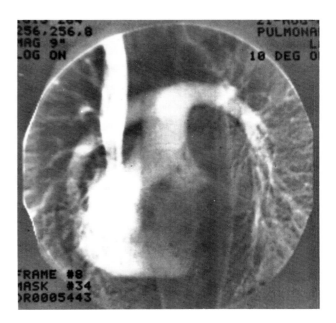
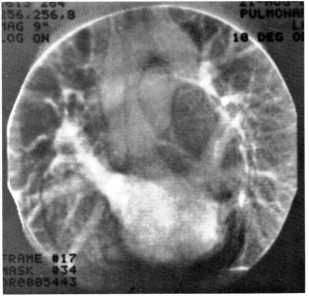
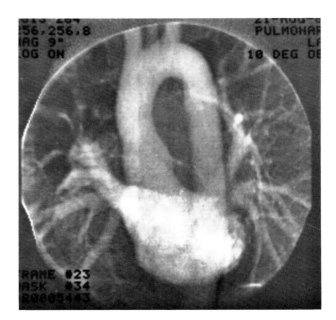

Fig. 112. Digital subtraction angiography of the heart

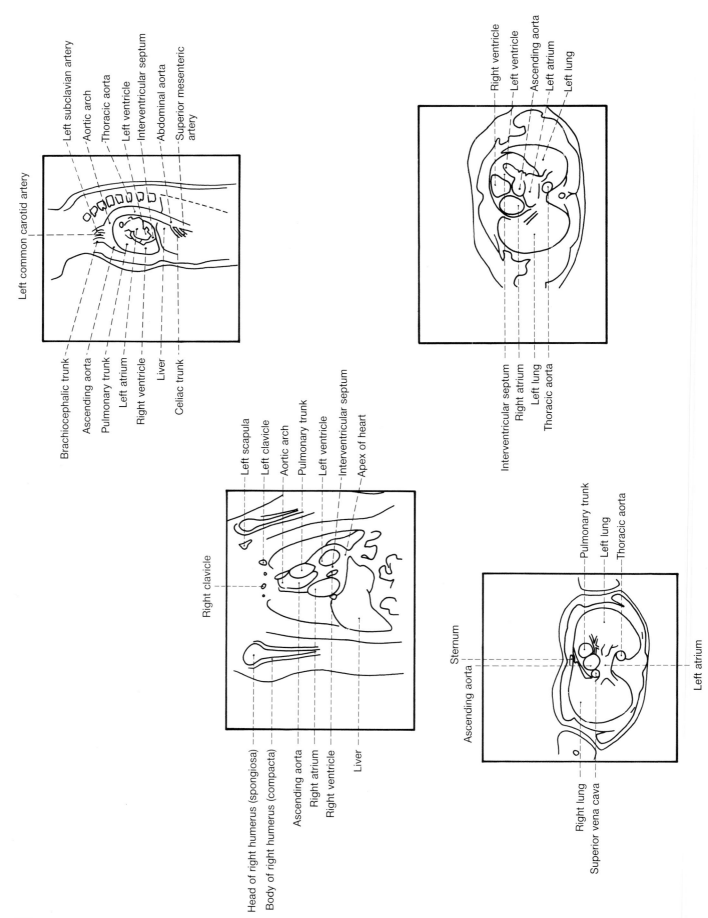

ERRATUM

Figs. 113a and b are turned
the wrong way. The diagrams
on page 178 are correct.

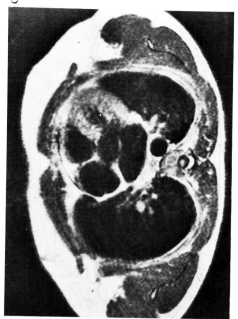

d

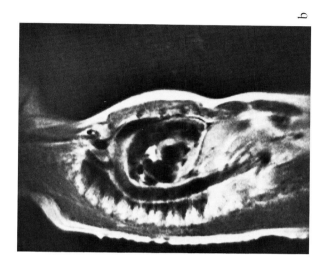

b

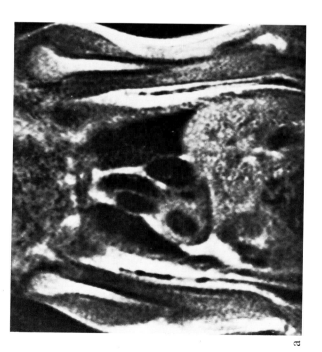

a

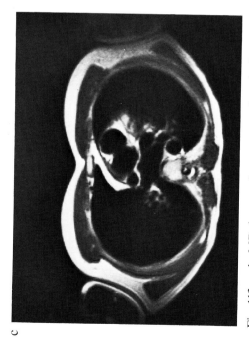

c

Fig. 113a–d. MR (magnetic resonance imaging) of the heart in frontal (coronal), sagittal (paramedian) and transverse (axial) sections

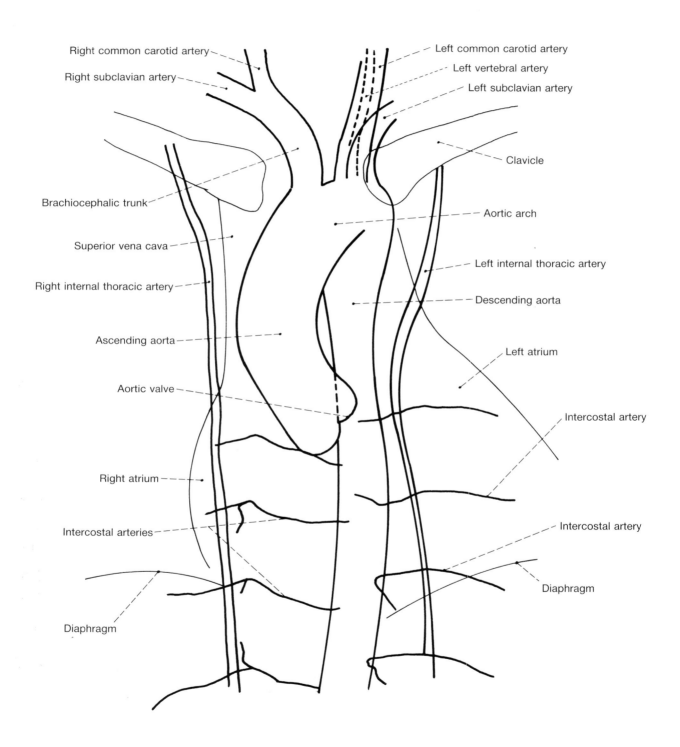

Right common carotid artery

Right subclavian artery

Left common carotid artery

Left vertebral artery

Left subclavian artery

Clavicle

Brachiocephalic trunk

Aortic arch

Superior vena cava

Left internal thoracic artery

Right internal thoracic artery

Descending aorta

Ascending aorta

Left atrium

Aortic valve

Intercostal artery

Right atrium

Intercostal artery

Intercostal arteries

Diaphragm

Diaphragm

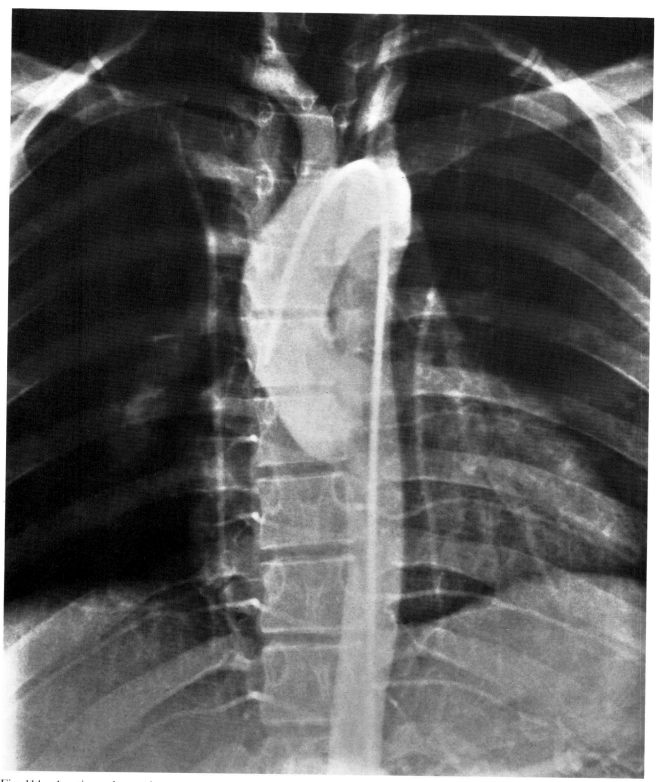

Fig. 114. Aortic arch, angiogram

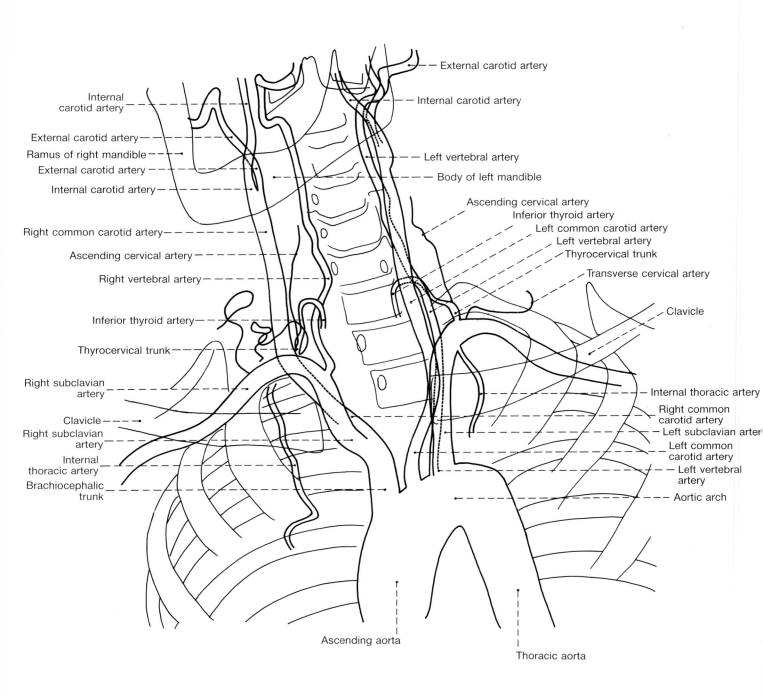

External carotid artery

Internal carotid artery

Internal carotid artery

External carotid artery

Ramus of right mandible

External carotid artery

Internal carotid artery

Left vertebral artery

Body of left mandible

Right common carotid artery

Ascending cervical artery

Right vertebral artery

Inferior thyroid artery

Thyrocervical trunk

Right subclavian artery

Clavicle

Right subclavian artery

Internal thoracic artery

Brachiocephalic trunk

Ascending cervical artery

Inferior thyroid artery

Left common carotid artery

Left vertebral artery

Thyrocervical trunk

Transverse cervical artery

Clavicle

Internal thoracic artery

Right common carotid artery

Left subclavian artery

Left common carotid artery

Left vertebral artery

Aortic arch

Ascending aorta

Thoracic aorta

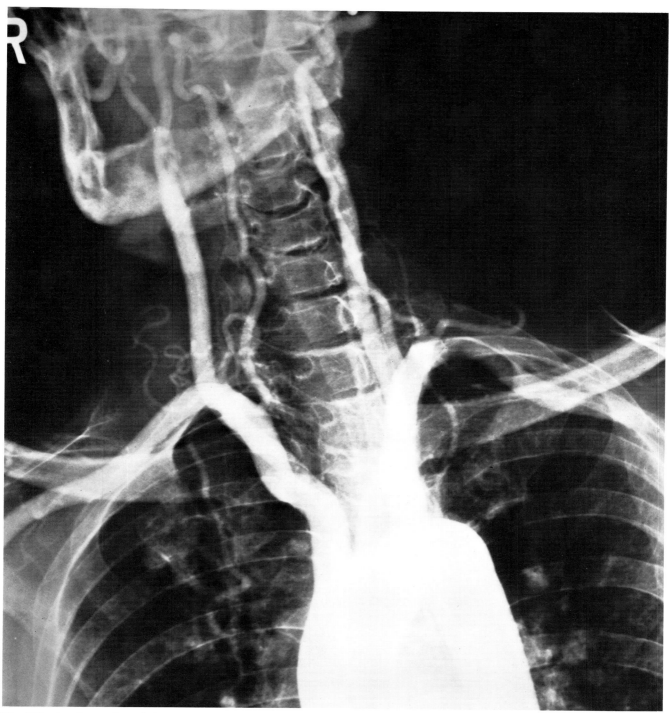

Fig. 115. Angiography of the aortic arch with its great vessels

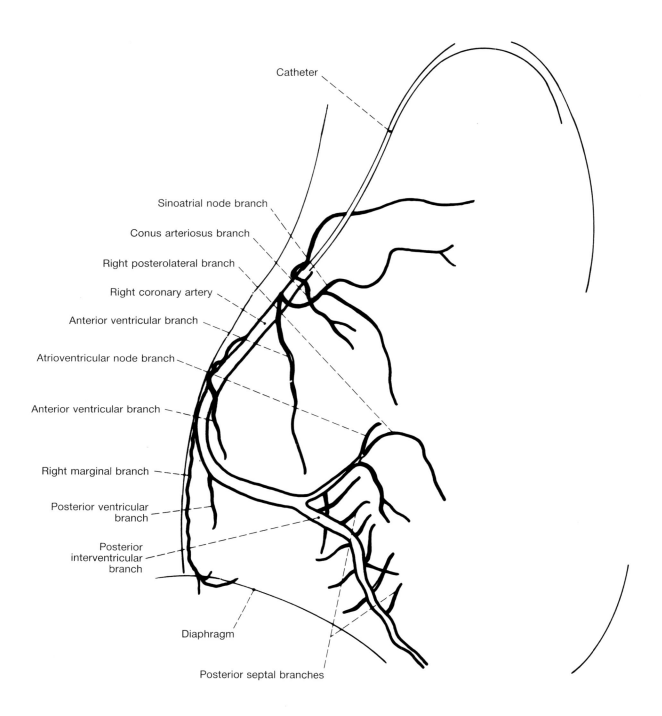

Catheter

Sinoatrial node branch

Conus arteriosus branch

Right posterolateral branch

Right coronary artery

Anterior ventricular branch

Atrioventricular node branch

Anterior ventricular branch

Right marginal branch

Posterior ventricular branch

Posterior interventricular branch

Diaphragm

Posterior septal branches

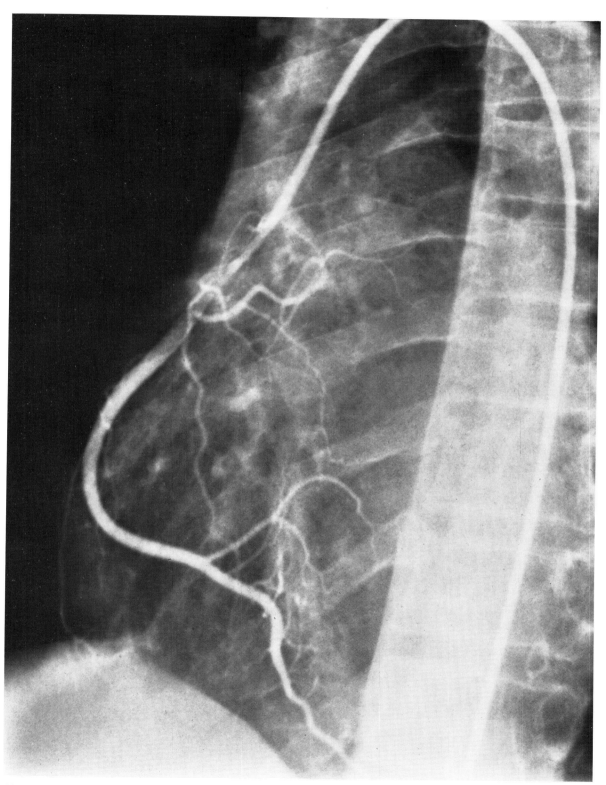

Fig. 116. Right coronary angiogram, left anterior oblique view

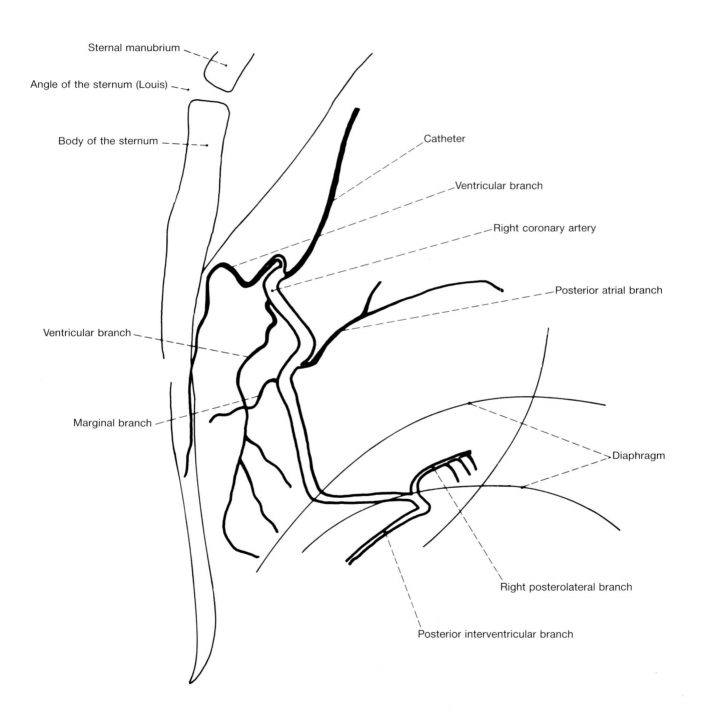

Sternal manubrium

Angle of the sternum (Louis)

Body of the sternum

Catheter

Ventricular branch

Right coronary artery

Posterior atrial branch

Ventricular branch

Marginal branch

Diaphragm

Right posterolateral branch

Posterior interventricular branch

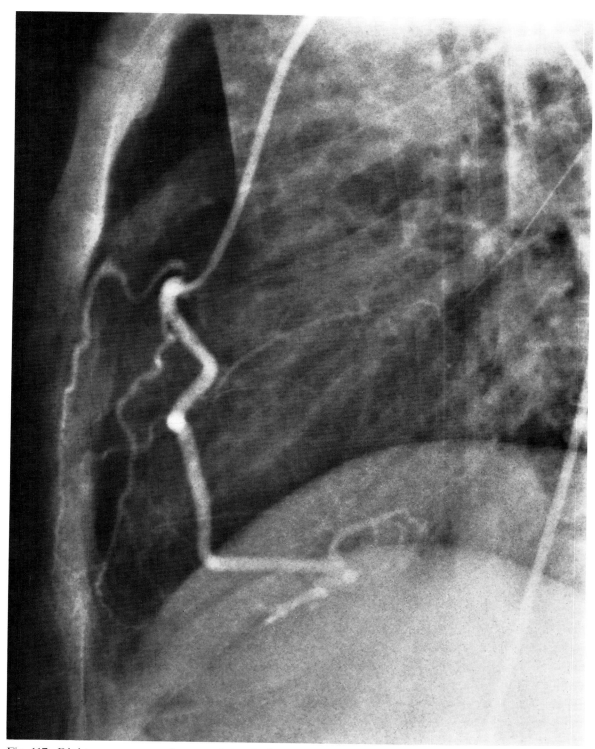

Fig. 117. Right coronary angiogram, lateral view

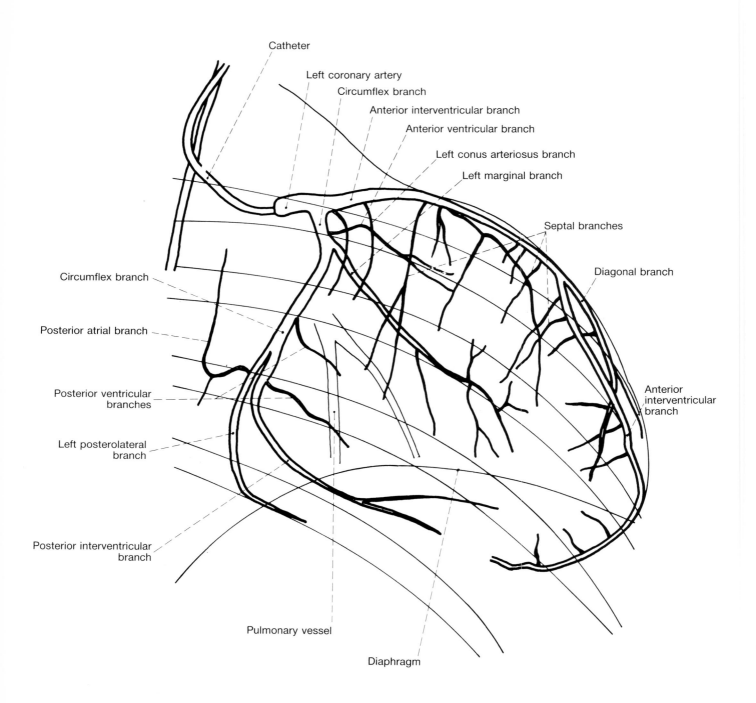

Catheter

Left coronary artery

Circumflex branch

Anterior interventricular branch

Anterior ventricular branch

Left conus arteriosus branch

Left marginal branch

Septal branches

Diagonal branch

Circumflex branch

Posterior atrial branch

Anterior interventricular branch

Posterior ventricular branches

Left posterolateral branch

Posterior interventricular branch

Pulmonary vessel

Diaphragm

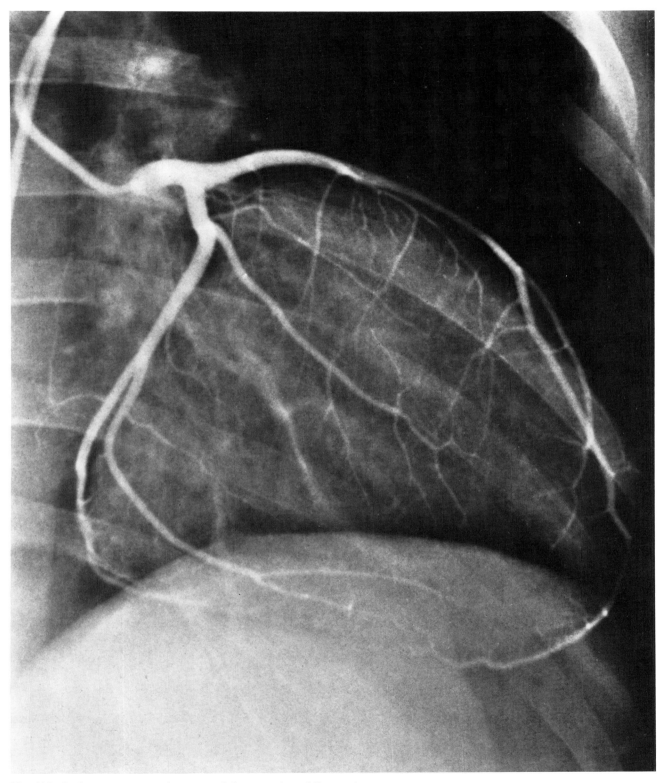

Fig. 118. Left coronary angiogram, right anterior oblique view

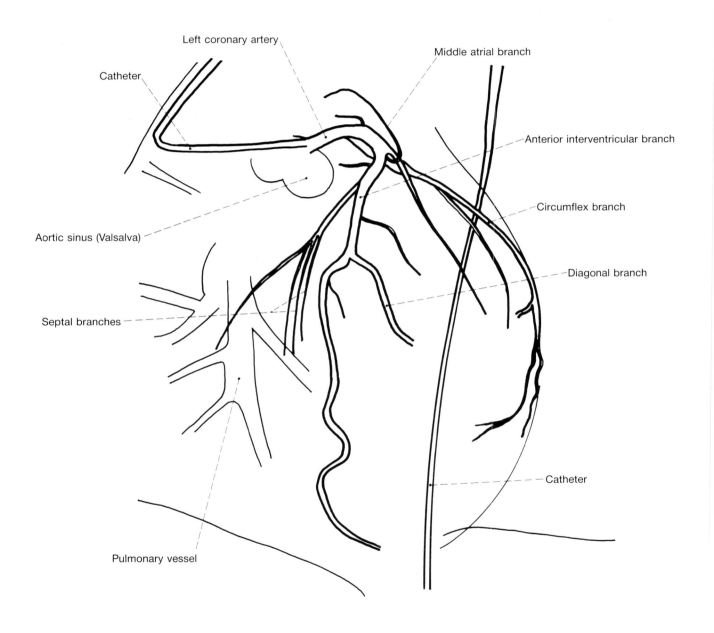

Left coronary artery

Catheter

Middle atrial branch

Anterior interventricular branch

Aortic sinus (Valsalva)

Circumflex branch

Diagonal branch

Septal branches

Catheter

Pulmonary vessel

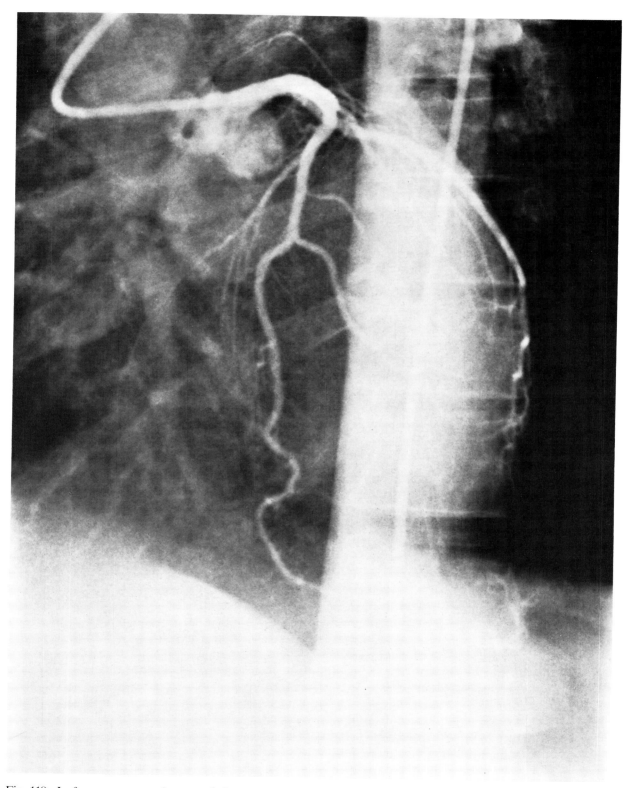

Fig. 119. Left coronary angiogram, left anterior oblique view

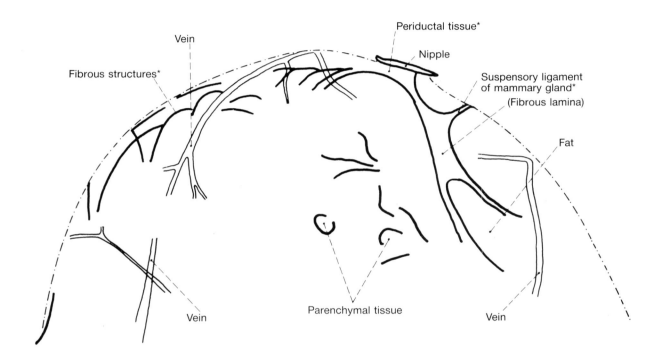

Vein

Fibrous structures*

Periductal tissue*

Nipple

Suspensory ligament
of mammary gland*
(Fibrous lamina)

Fat

Vein

Parenchymal tissue

Vein

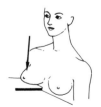

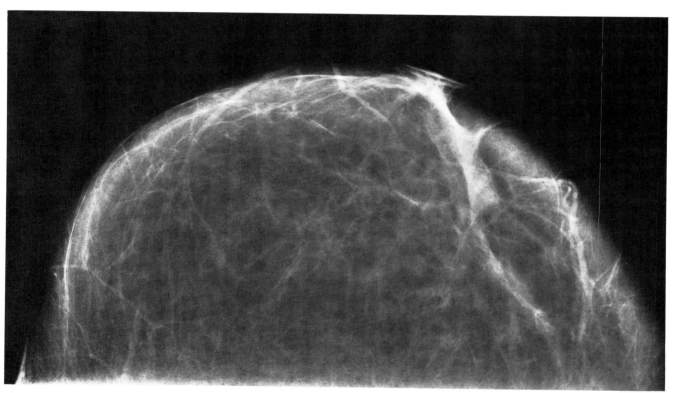

Fig. 120. Mammogram, craniocaudal view

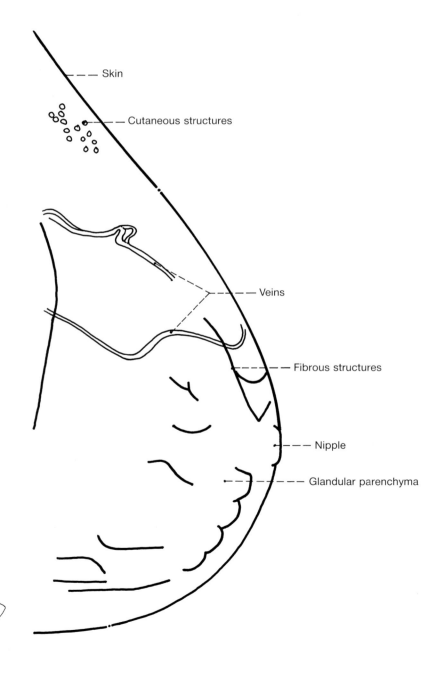

Skin

Cutaneous structures

Veins

Fibrous structures

Nipple

Glandular parenchyma

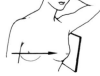

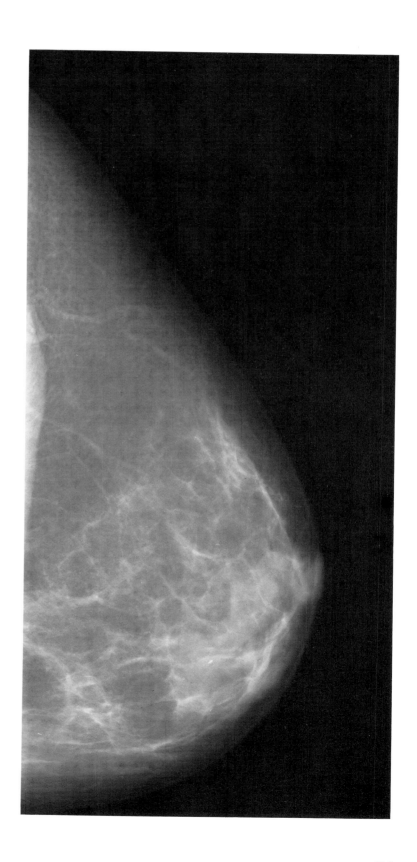

Fig. 121. Mammogram, lateral view

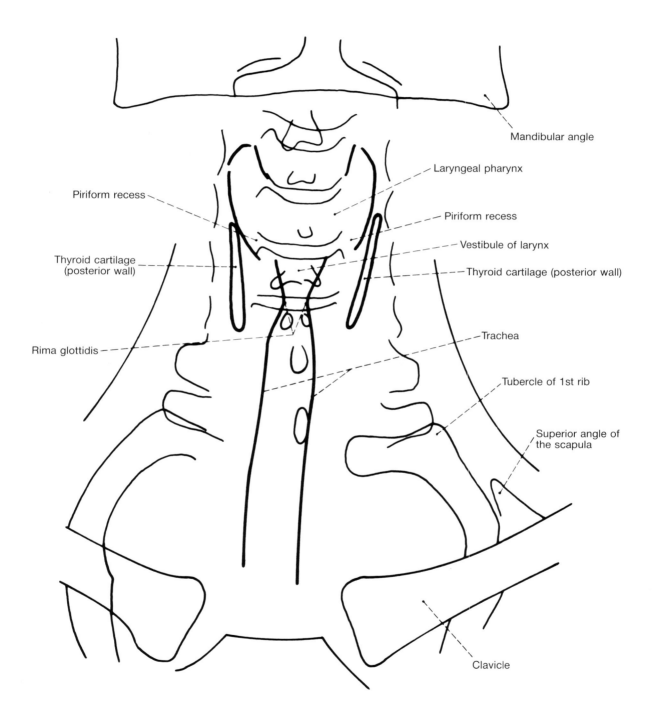

Mandibular angle

Laryngeal pharynx

Piriform recess

Piriform recess

Vestibule of larynx

Thyroid cartilage
(posterior wall)

Thyroid cartilage (posterior wall)

Trachea

Rima glottidis

Tubercle of 1st rib

Superior angle of
the scapula

Clavicle

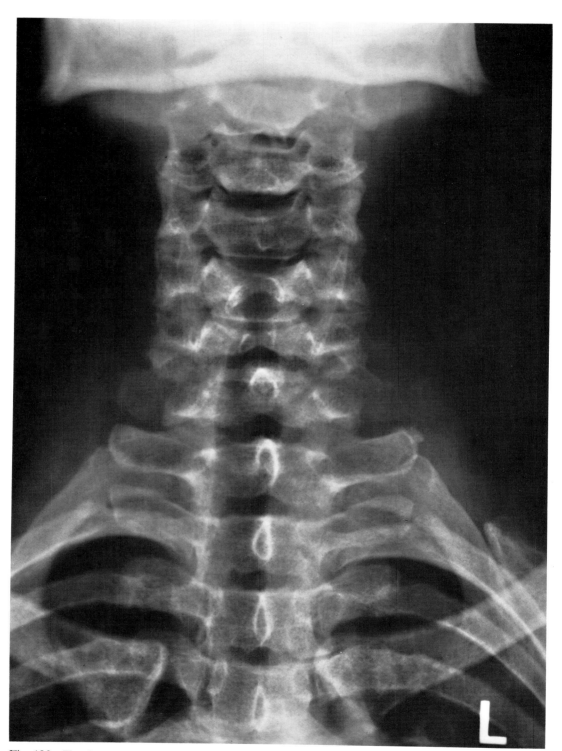

Fig. 122. Trachea, p.a. view

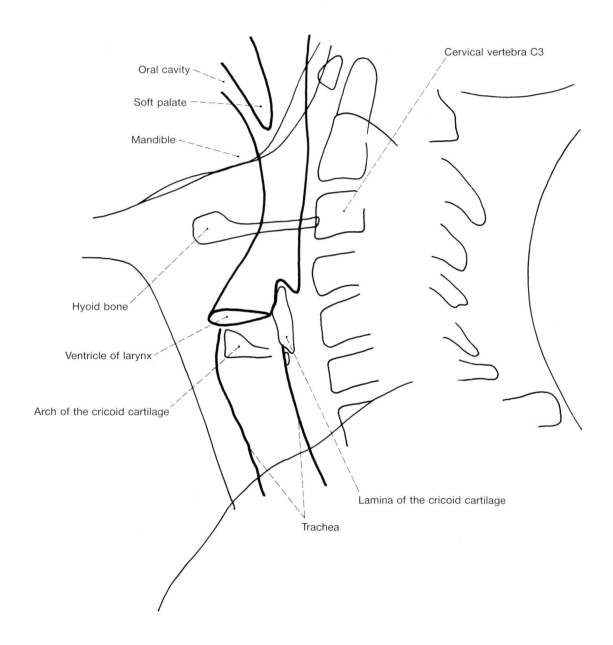

Oral cavity

Soft palate

Mandible

Cervical vertebra C3

Hyoid bone

Ventricle of larynx

Arch of the cricoid cartilage

Lamina of the cricoid cartilage

Trachea

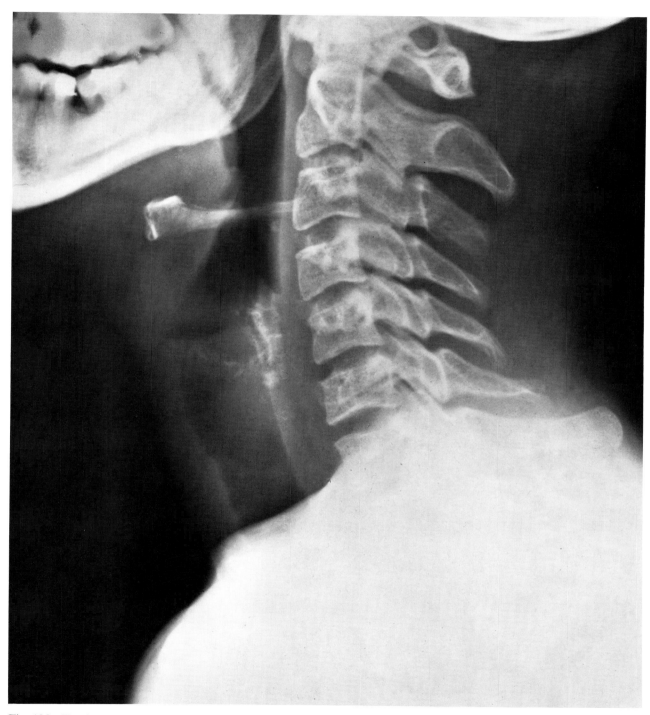

Fig. 123. Trachea, lateral view

Digestive Tract

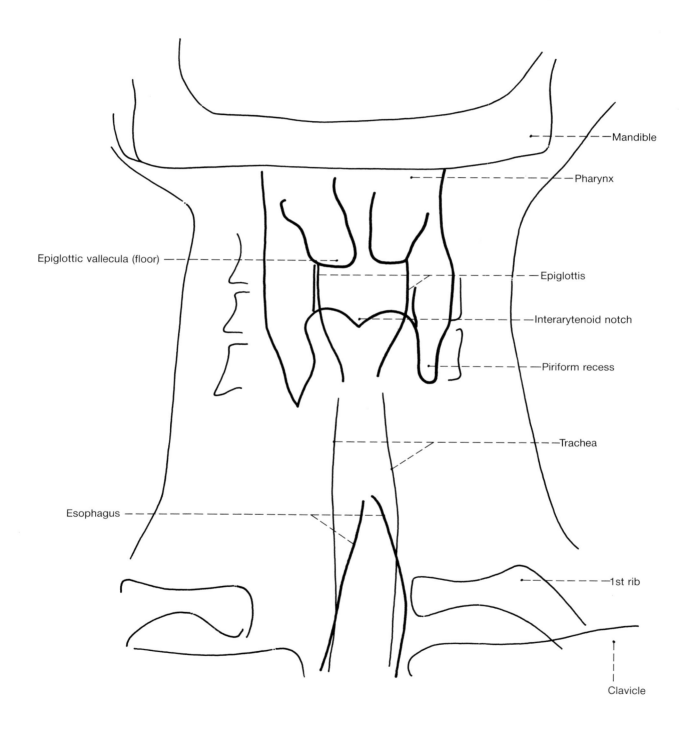

Mandible

Pharynx

Epiglottic vallecula (floor)

Epiglottis

Interarytenoid notch

Piriform recess

Trachea

Esophagus

1st rib

Clavicle

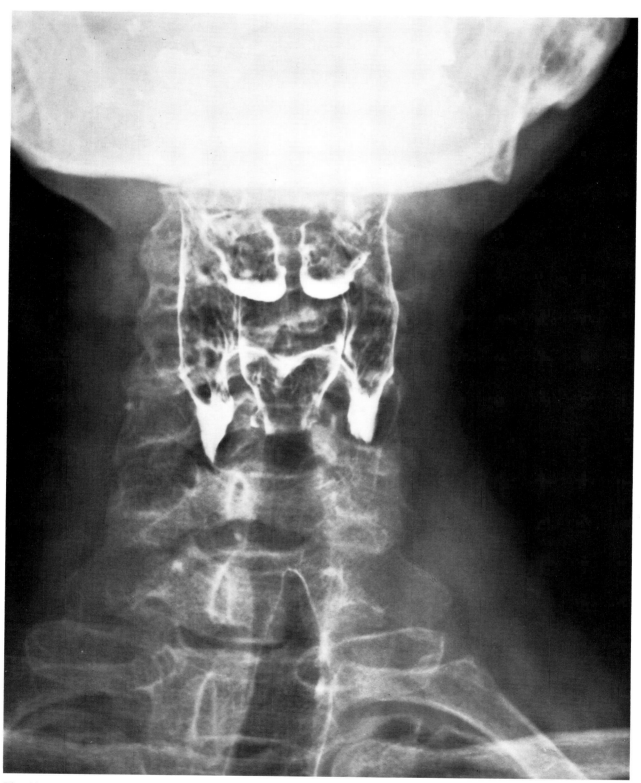

Fig. 124. Deglutition, p.a. view

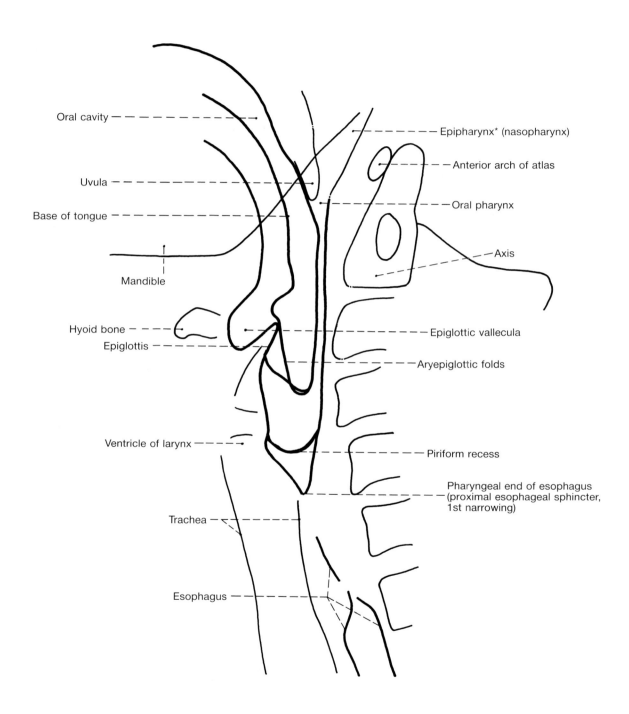

Oral cavity – – – – – – – – – –

Epipharynx* (nasopharynx)

Anterior arch of atlas

Uvula – – – – – – – – – – – –

Base of tongue – – – – – – – – –

Oral pharynx

Axis

Mandible

Hyoid bone – – – –

Epiglottic vallecula

Epiglottis – – – – – –

Aryepiglottic folds

Ventricle of larynx – – – – – –

Piriform recess

Pharyngeal end of esophagus
(proximal esophageal sphincter,
1st narrowing)

Trachea – – – –

Esophagus – – – – –

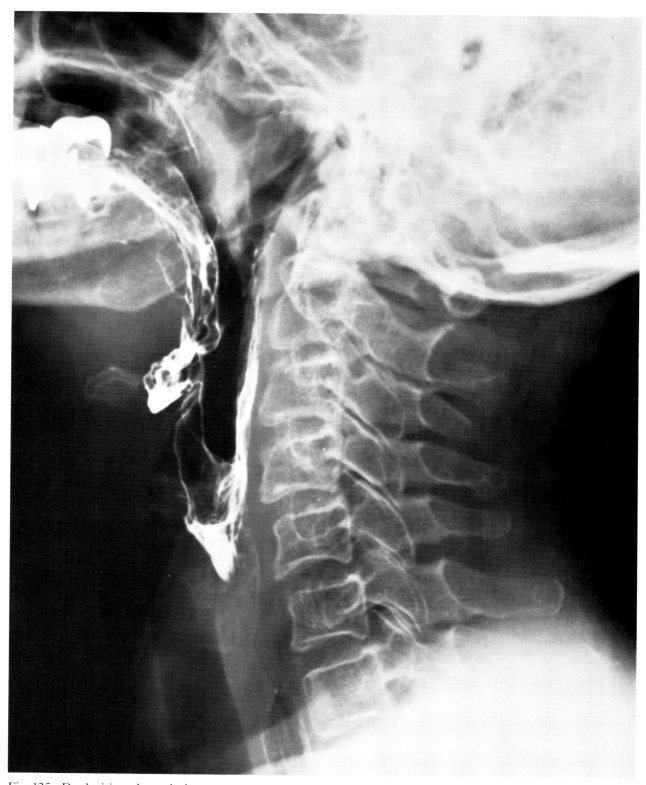

Fig. 125. Deglutition, lateral view

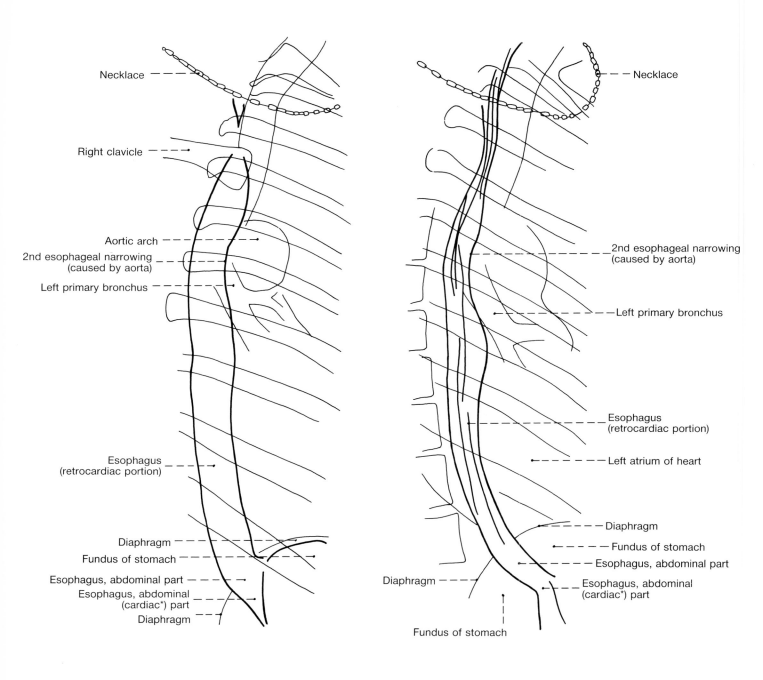

Necklace

Right clavicle

Aortic arch

2nd esophageal narrowing
(caused by aorta)

Left primary bronchus

Esophagus
(retrocardiac portion)

Diaphragm

Fundus of stomach

Esophagus, abdominal part

Esophagus, abdominal
(cardiac*) part

Diaphragm

Necklace

2nd esophageal narrowing
(caused by aorta)

Left primary bronchus

Esophagus
(retrocardiac portion)

Left atrium of heart

Diaphragm

Fundus of stomach

Esophagus, abdominal part

Esophagus, abdominal
(cardiac*) part

Diaphragm

Fundus of stomach

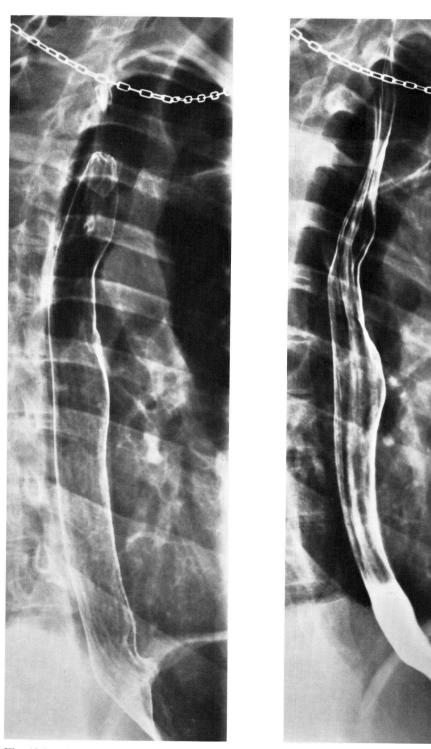

Fig. 126a. Esophagus, two right anterior oblique views

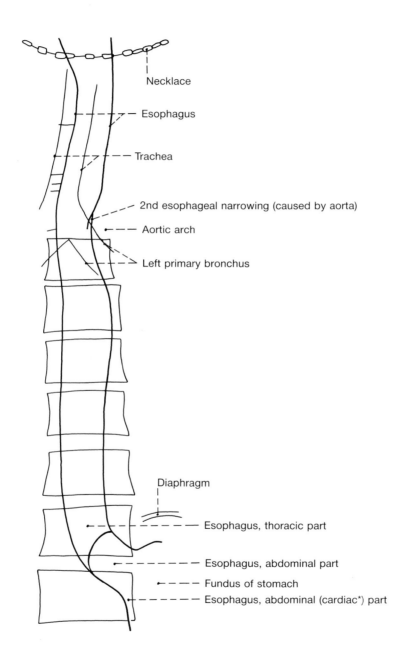

Necklace

Esophagus

Trachea

2nd esophageal narrowing (caused by aorta)

Aortic arch

Left primary bronchus

Diaphragm

Esophagus, thoracic part

Esophagus, abdominal part

Fundus of stomach

Esophagus, abdominal (cardiac*) part

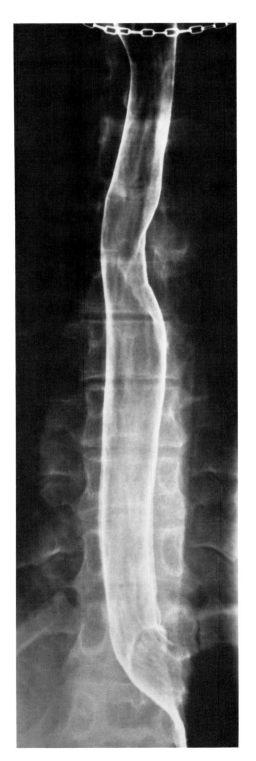

Fig. 126b. Esophagus, p.a. view

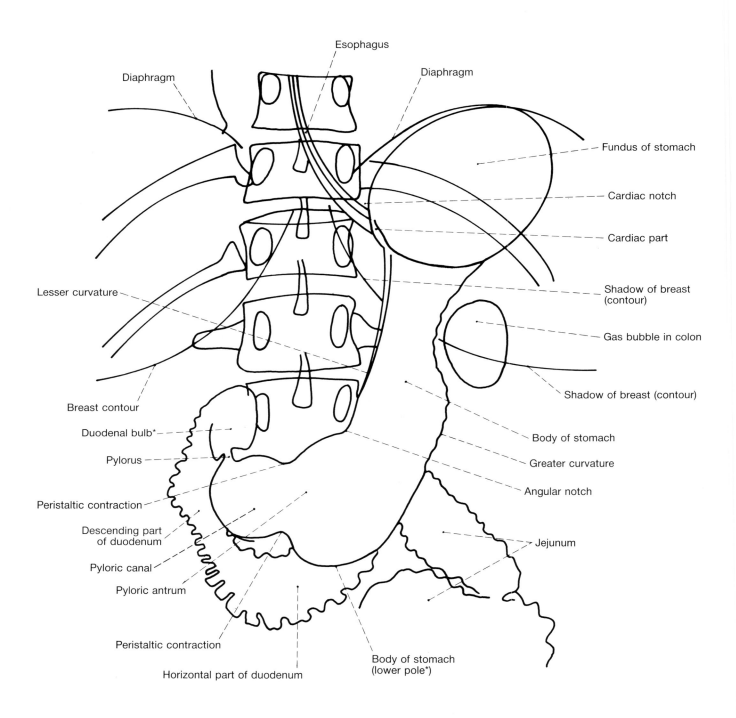

Esophagus

Diaphragm

Diaphragm

Fundus of stomach

Cardiac notch

Cardiac part

Shadow of breast
(contour)

Gas bubble in colon

Lesser curvature

Shadow of breast (contour)

Body of stomach

Greater curvature

Breast contour

Angular notch

Duodenal bulb*

Pylorus

Jejunum

Peristaltic contraction

Descending part
of duodenum

Pyloric canal

Pyloric antrum

Peristaltic contraction

Body of stomach
(lower pole*)

Horizontal part of duodenum

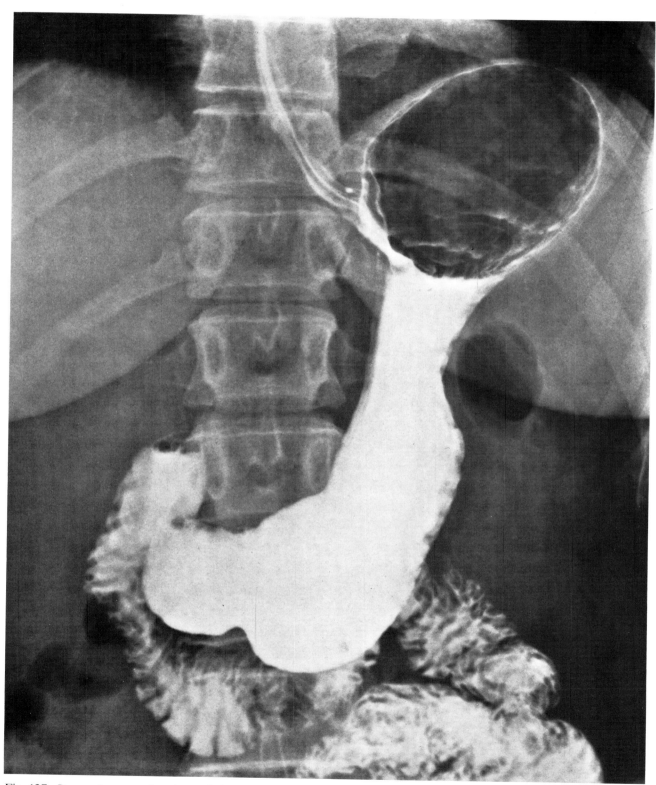

Fig. 127. Stomach, p.a. view in upright position (J-shaped)

Stomach

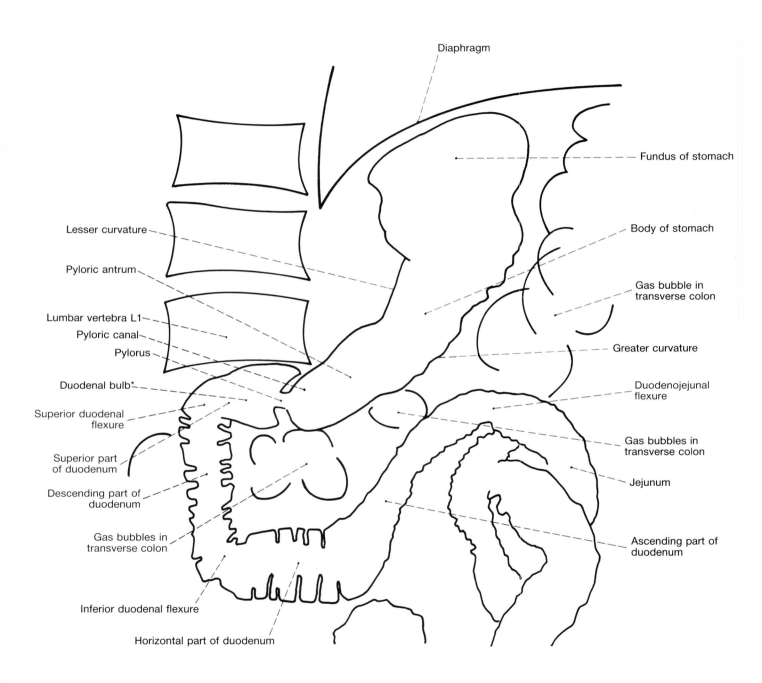

Diaphragm

Fundus of stomach

Body of stomach

Gas bubble in
transverse colon

Greater curvature

Duodenojejunal
flexure

Gas bubbles in
transverse colon

Jejunum

Ascending part of
duodenum

Lesser curvature

Pyloric antrum

Lumbar vertebra L1

Pyloric canal

Pylorus

Duodenal bulb*

Superior duodenal
flexure

Superior part
of duodenum

Descending part of
duodenum

Gas bubbles in
transverse colon

Inferior duodenal flexure

Horizontal part of duodenum

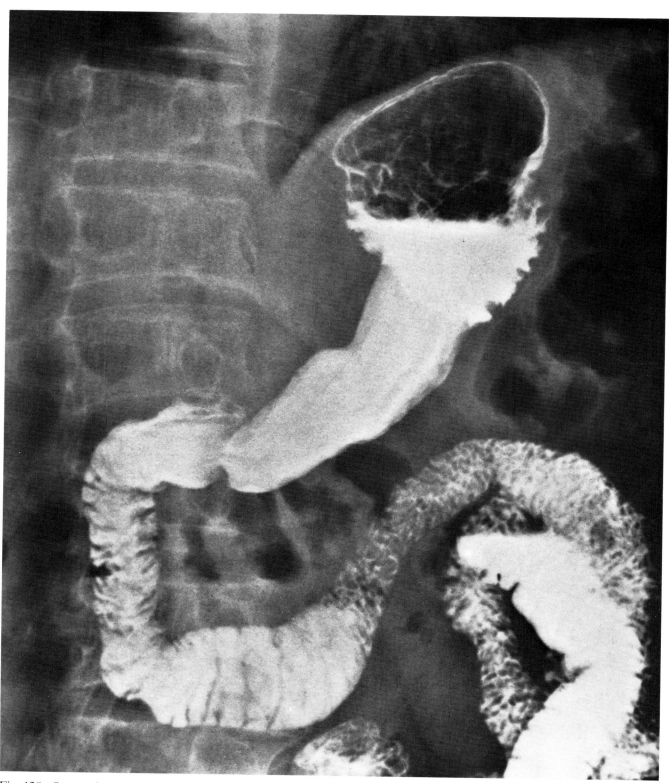

Fig. 128. Stomach, p.a. view in upright position

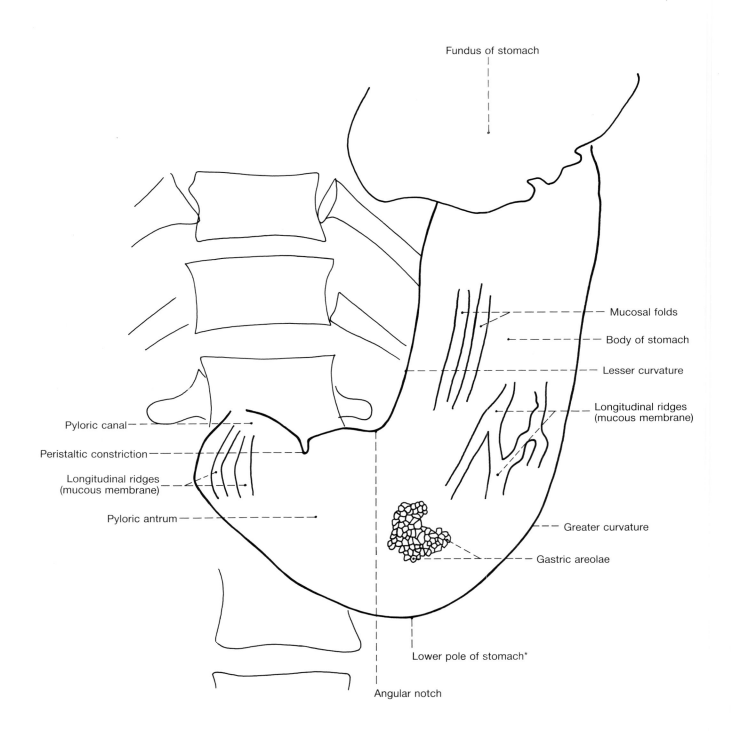

Fundus of stomach

Mucosal folds

Body of stomach

Lesser curvature

Longitudinal ridges
(mucous membrane)

Pyloric canal

Peristaltic constriction

Longitudinal ridges
(mucous membrane)

Pyloric antrum

Greater curvature

Gastric areolae

Lower pole of stomach*

Angular notch

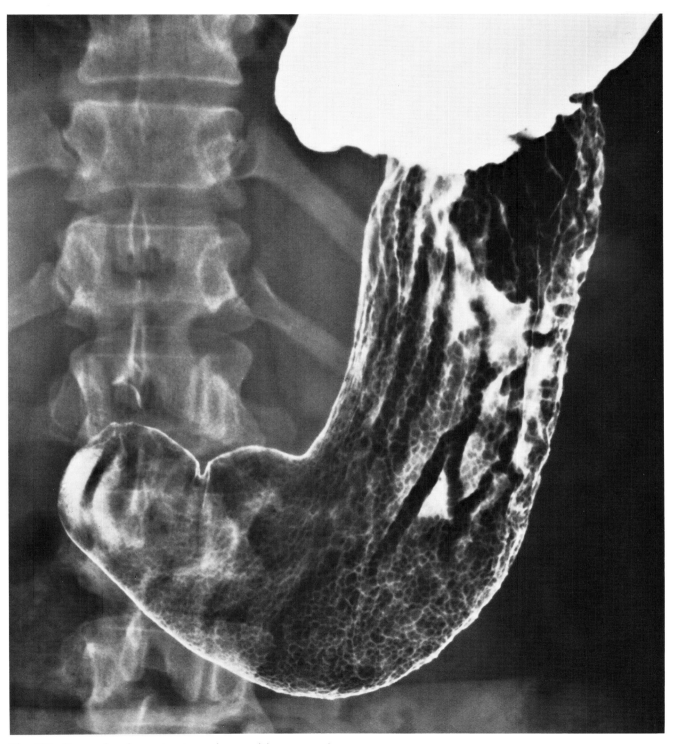

Fig. 129. Stomach, air contrast, supine position, p.a. view

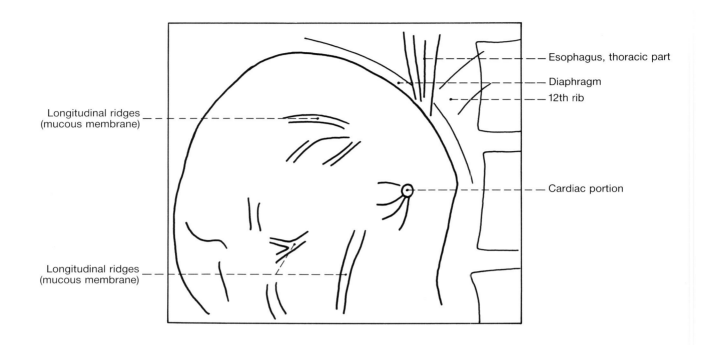

Esophagus, thoracic part

Diaphragm

12th rib

Longitudinal ridges
(mucous membrane)

Cardiac portion

Longitudinal ridges
(mucous membrane)

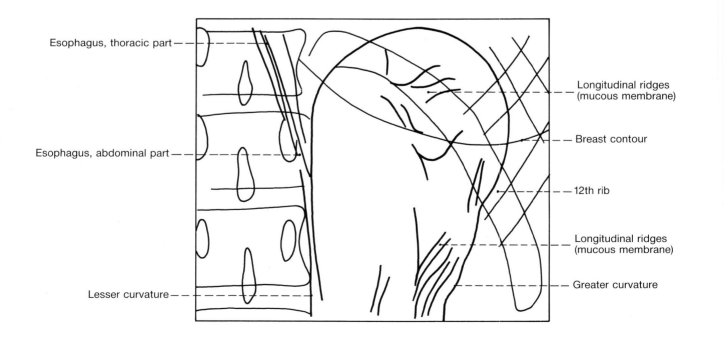

Esophagus, thoracic part

Longitudinal ridges
(mucous membrane)

Breast contour

Esophagus, abdominal part

12th rib

Longitudinal ridges
(mucous membrane)

Lesser curvature

Greater curvature

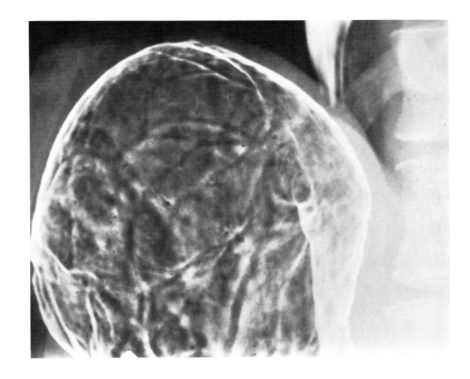

Fig. 130. Fundus of stomach, a.p. coned-down image in prone position (right anterior oblique view)

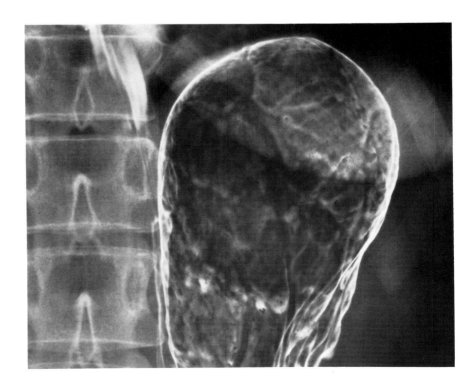

Fig. 131. Fundus of stomach, p.a. coned-down image in upright position

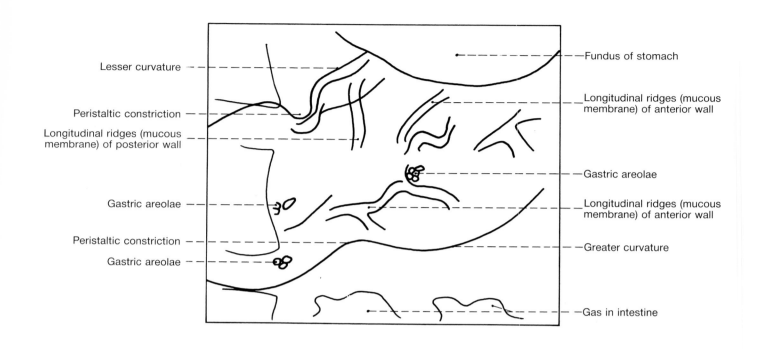

Lesser curvature

Peristaltic constriction

Longitudinal ridges (mucous membrane) of posterior wall

Gastric areolae

Peristaltic constriction

Gastric areolae

Fundus of stomach

Longitudinal ridges (mucous membrane) of anterior wall

Gastric areolae

Longitudinal ridges (mucous membrane) of anterior wall

Greater curvature

Gas in intestine

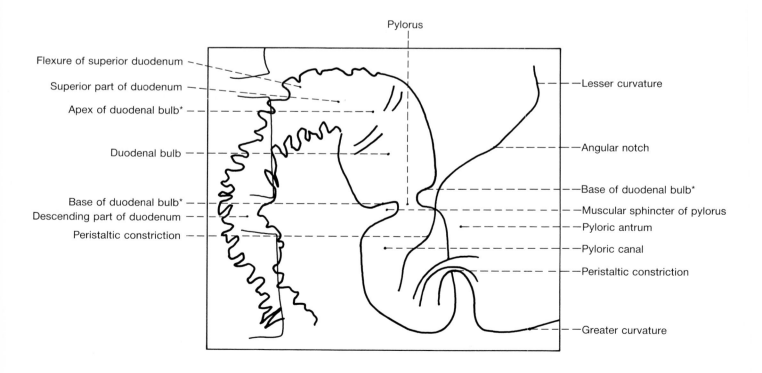

Pylorus

Flexure of superior duodenum

Superior part of duodenum

Apex of duodenal bulb*

Duodenal bulb

Base of duodenal bulb*

Descending part of duodenum

Peristaltic constriction

Lesser curvature

Angular notch

Base of duodenal bulb*

Muscular sphincter of pylorus

Pyloric antrum

Pyloric canal

Peristaltic constriction

Greater curvature

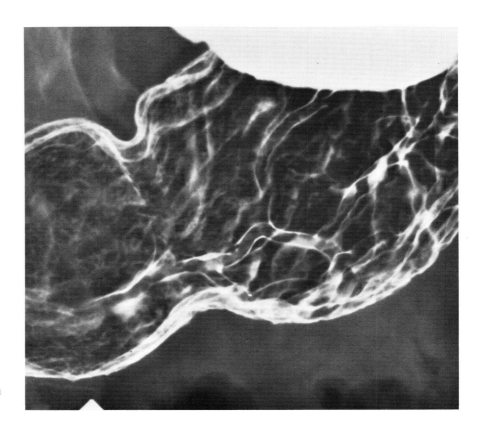

Fig. 132. Stomach, p.a. coned-down image in supine position

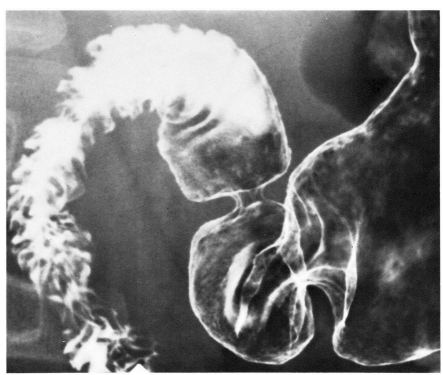

Fig. 133. Pyloric part and duodenal bulb, p.a. coned-down image in supine position (right anterior oblique view)

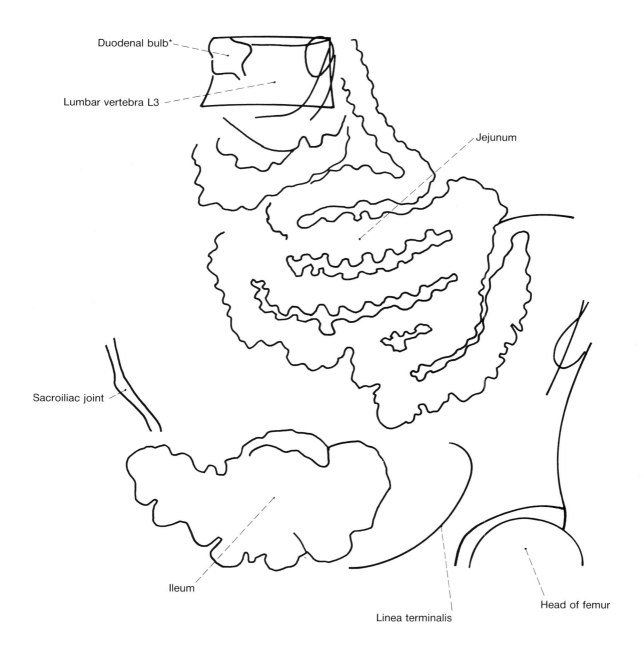

Duodenal bulb*

Lumbar vertebra L3

Jejunum

Sacroiliac joint

Ileum

Linea terminalis

Head of femur

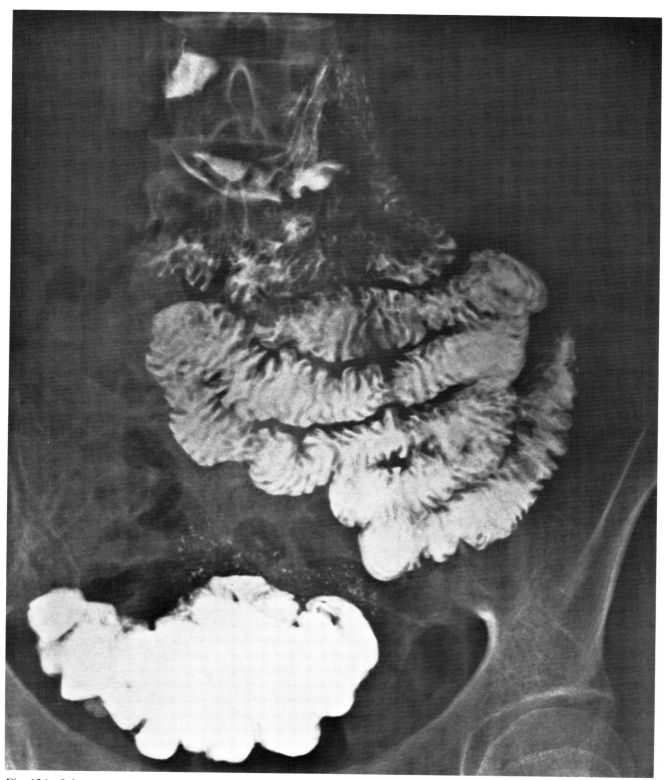

Fig. 134. Jejunum and ileum

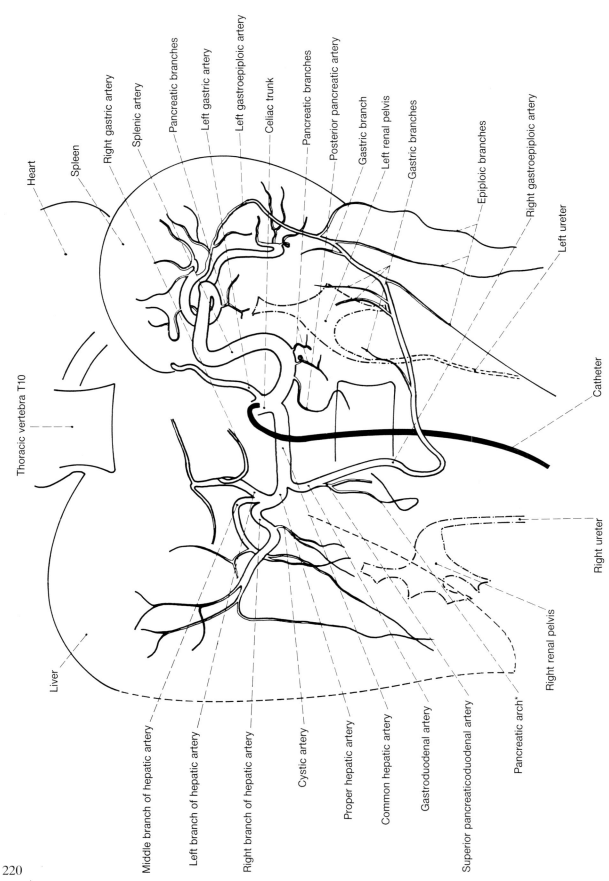

Heart

Spleen

Right gastric artery

Splenic artery

Pancreatic branches

Left gastric artery

Left gastroepiploic artery

Celiac trunk

Pancreatic branches

Posterior pancreatic artery

Gastric branch

Left renal pelvis

Gastric branches

Epiploic branches

Right gastroepiploic artery

Left ureter

Catheter

Thoracic vertebra T10

Right ureter

Right renal pelvis

Pancreatic arch*

Superior pancreaticoduodenal artery

Gastroduodenal artery

Common hepatic artery

Proper hepatic artery

Cystic artery

Right branch of hepatic artery

Left branch of hepatic artery

Middle branch of hepatic artery

Liver

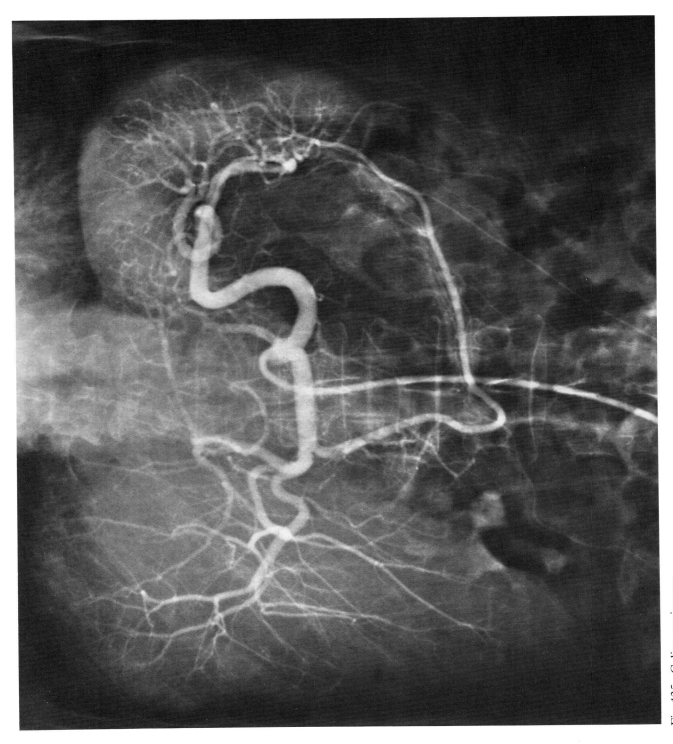

Fig. 135. Celiac angiogram

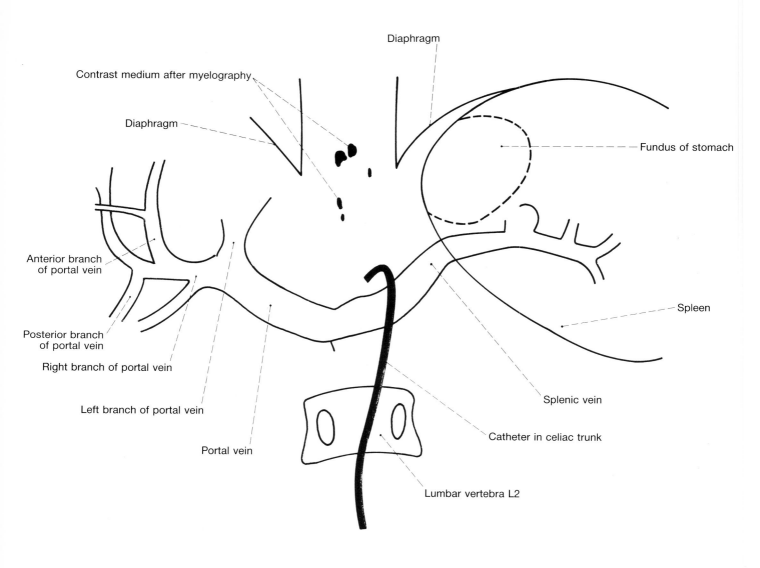

Diaphragm

Contrast medium after myelography

Diaphragm

Fundus of stomach

Anterior branch
of portal vein

Spleen

Posterior branch
of portal vein

Right branch of portal vein

Splenic vein

Left branch of portal vein

Catheter in celiac trunk

Portal vein

Lumbar vertebra L2

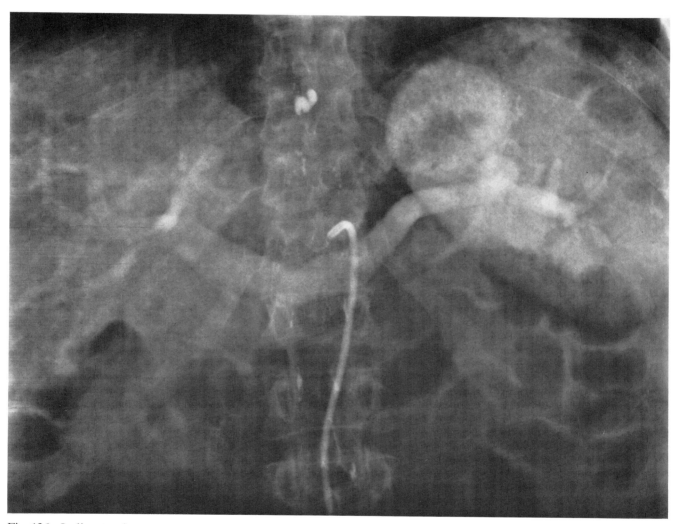

Fig. 136. Indirect splenoportogram

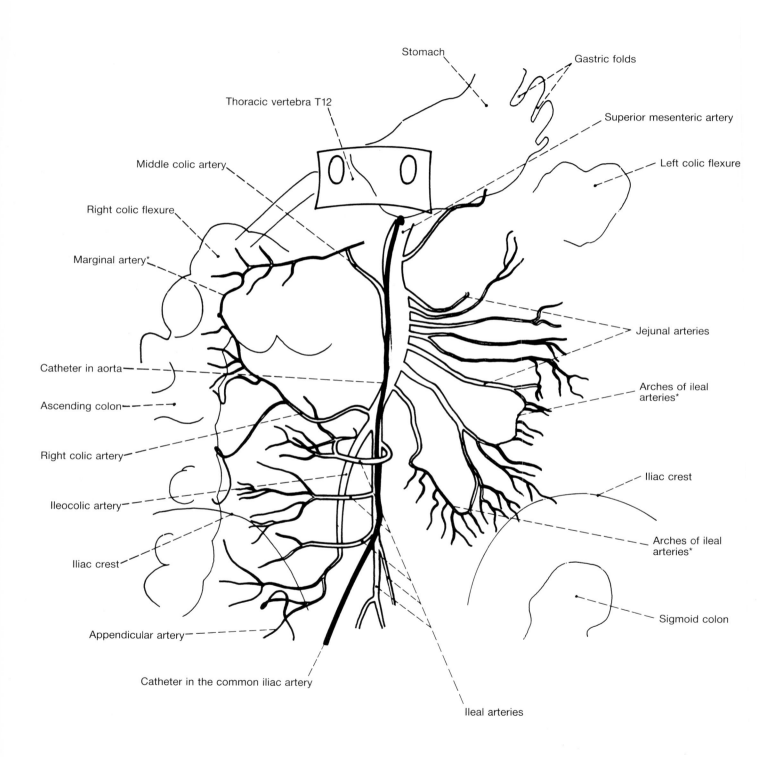

Stomach

Gastric folds

Thoracic vertebra T12

Superior mesenteric artery

Middle colic artery

Left colic flexure

Right colic flexure

Marginal artery*

Jejunal arteries

Catheter in aorta

Arches of ileal arteries*

Ascending colon

Right colic artery

Iliac crest

Ileocolic artery

Arches of ileal arteries*

Iliac crest

Appendicular artery

Sigmoid colon

Catheter in the common iliac artery

Ileal arteries

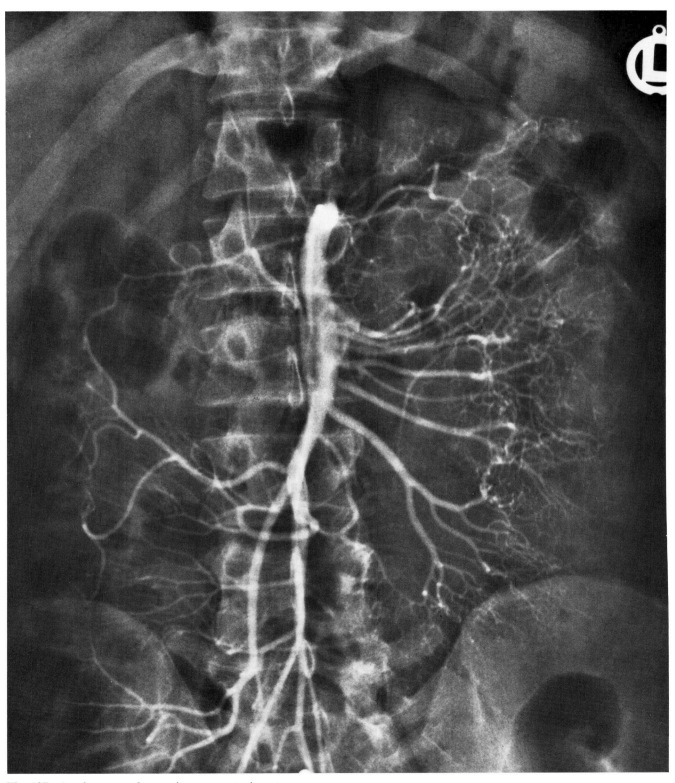

Fig. 137. Angiogram of superior mesenteric artery

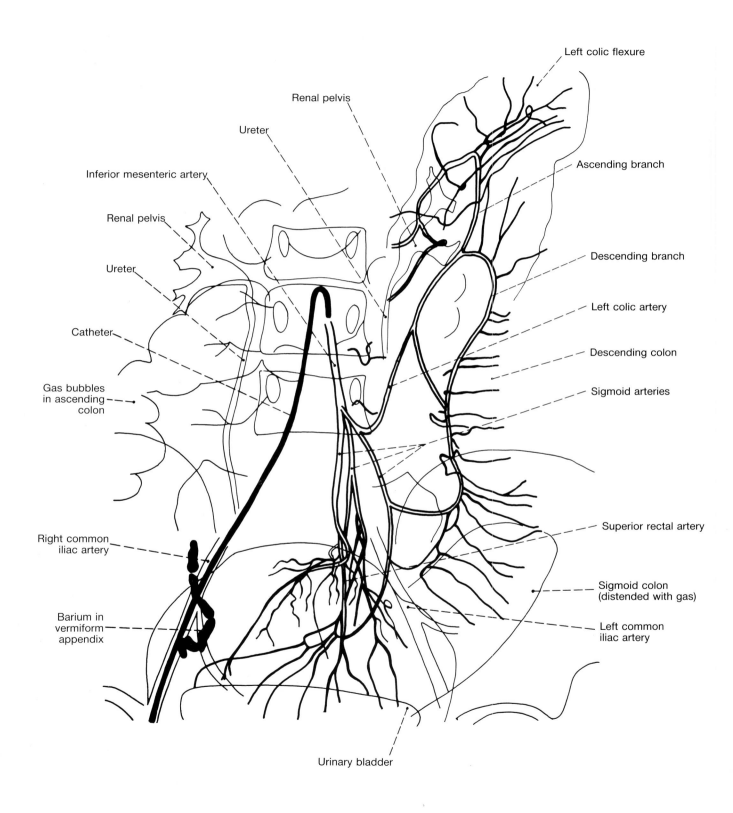

Left colic flexure

Renal pelvis

Ureter

Ascending branch

Inferior mesenteric artery

Renal pelvis

Descending branch

Left colic artery

Ureter

Descending colon

Catheter

Sigmoid arteries

Gas bubbles
in ascending
colon

Superior rectal artery

Right common
iliac artery

Sigmoid colon
(distended with gas)

Barium in
vermiform
appendix

Left common
iliac artery

Urinary bladder

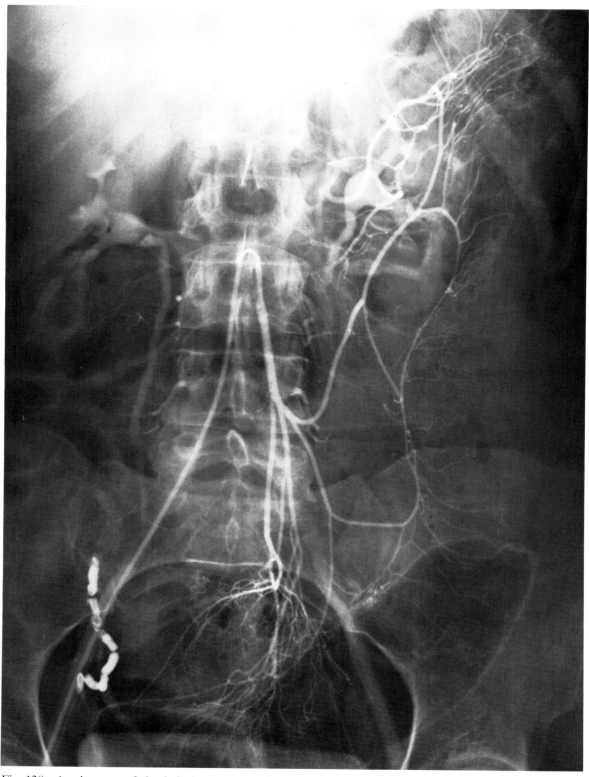

Fig. 138. Angiogram of the inferior mesenteric artery

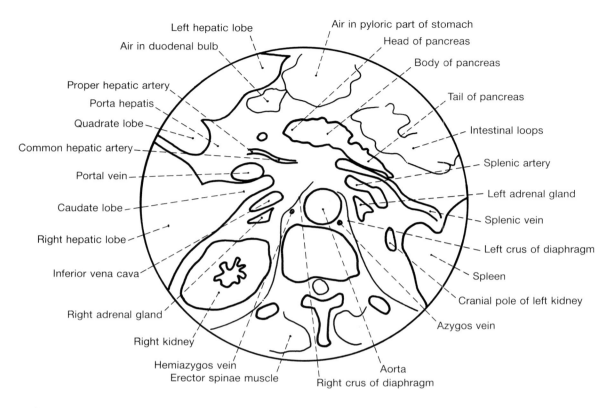

Left hepatic lobe
Air in duodenal bulb
Proper hepatic artery
Porta hepatis
Quadrate lobe
Common hepatic artery
Portal vein
Caudate lobe
Right hepatic lobe
Inferior vena cava
Right adrenal gland
Right kidney
Hemiazygos vein
Erector spinae muscle

Air in pyloric part of stomach
Head of pancreas
Body of pancreas
Tail of pancreas
Intestinal loops
Splenic artery
Left adrenal gland
Splenic vein
Left crus of diaphragm
Spleen
Cranial pole of left kidney
Azygos vein
Aorta
Right crus of diaphragm

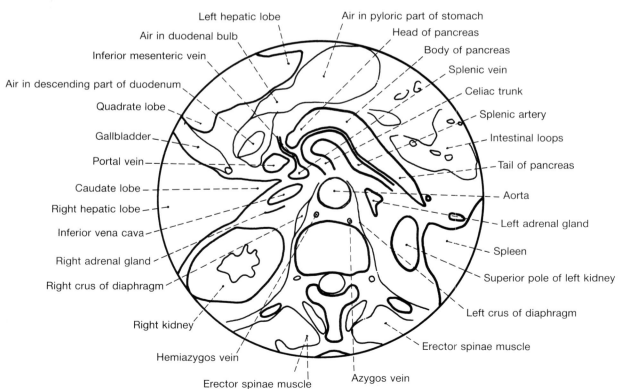

Left hepatic lobe
Air in duodenal bulb
Inferior mesenteric vein
Air in descending part of duodenum
Quadrate lobe
Gallbladder
Portal vein
Caudate lobe
Right hepatic lobe
Inferior vena cava
Right adrenal gland
Right crus of diaphragm
Right kidney
Hemiazygos vein
Erector spinae muscle

Air in pyloric part of stomach
Head of pancreas
Body of pancreas
Splenic vein
Celiac trunk
Splenic artery
Intestinal loops
Tail of pancreas
Aorta
Left adrenal gland
Spleen
Superior pole of left kidney
Left crus of diaphragm
Erector spinae muscle
Azygos vein

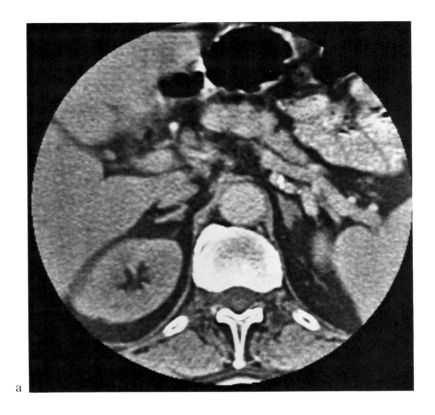

a

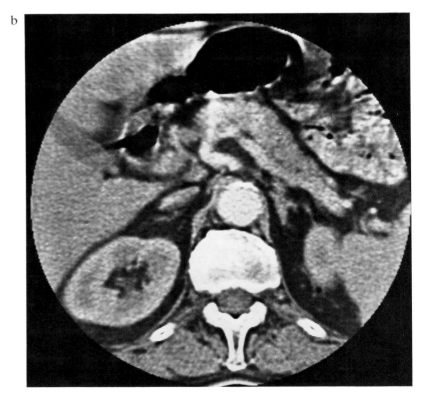

b

Fig. 139 a, b.
Computed axial tomograms of upper
abdomen (sectional views)

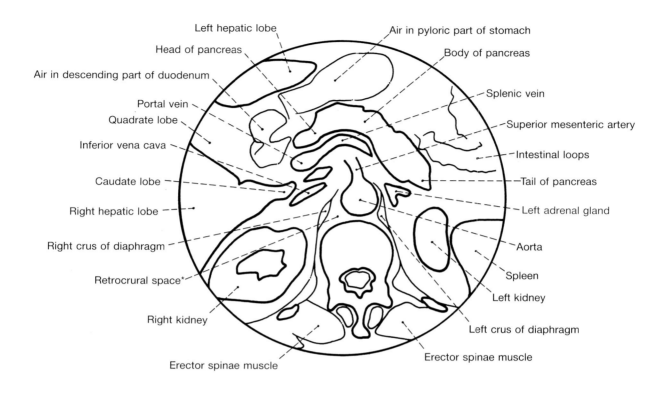

Left hepatic lobe

Head of pancreas

Air in descending part of duodenum

Portal vein

Quadrate lobe

Inferior vena cava

Caudate lobe

Right hepatic lobe

Right crus of diaphragm

Retrocrural space*

Right kidney

Erector spinae muscle

Air in pyloric part of stomach

Body of pancreas

Splenic vein

Superior mesenteric artery

Intestinal loops

Tail of pancreas

Left adrenal gland

Aorta

Spleen

Left kidney

Left crus of diaphragm

Erector spinae muscle

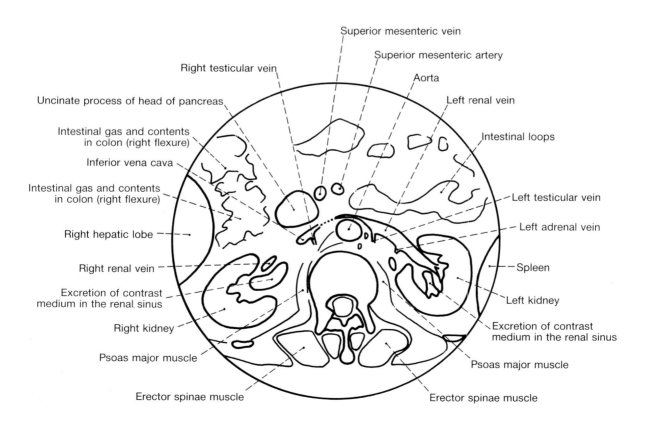

Superior mesenteric vein

Superior mesenteric artery

Aorta

Left renal vein

Right testicular vein

Uncinate process of head of pancreas

Intestinal gas and contents in colon (right flexure)

Inferior vena cava

Intestinal gas and contents in colon (right flexure)

Right hepatic lobe

Right renal vein

Excretion of contrast medium in the renal sinus

Right kidney

Psoas major muscle

Erector spinae muscle

Intestinal loops

Left testicular vein

Left adrenal vein

Spleen

Left kidney

Excretion of contrast medium in the renal sinus

Psoas major muscle

Erector spinae muscle

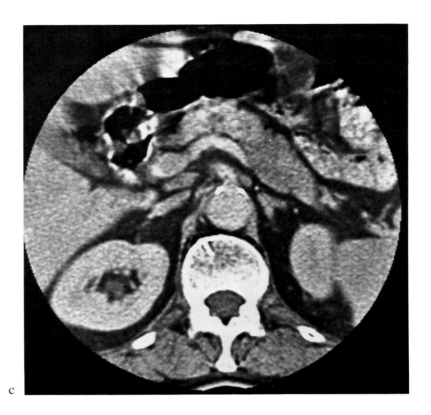

c

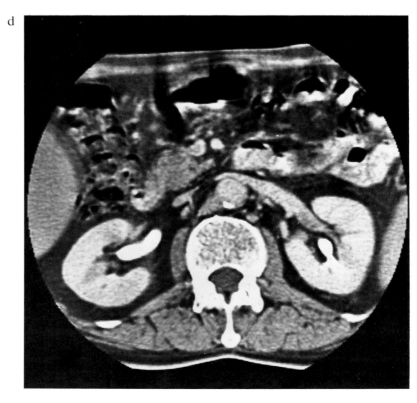

d

Fig. 139c, d.
Computed axial tomograms of upper
abdomen (sectional views)

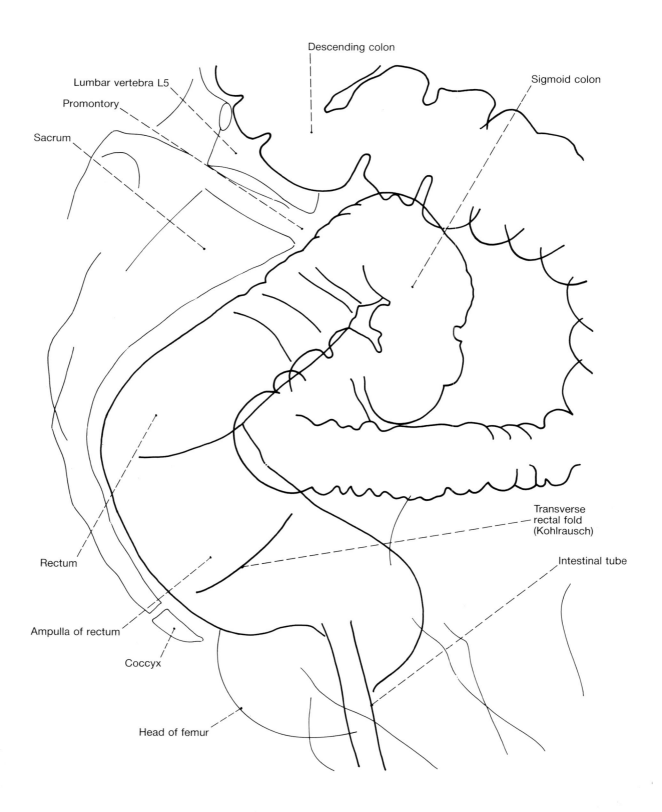

Descending colon

Sigmoid colon

Lumbar vertebra L5

Promontory

Sacrum

Transverse
rectal fold
(Kohlrausch)

Intestinal tube

Rectum

Ampulla of rectum

Coccyx

Head of femur

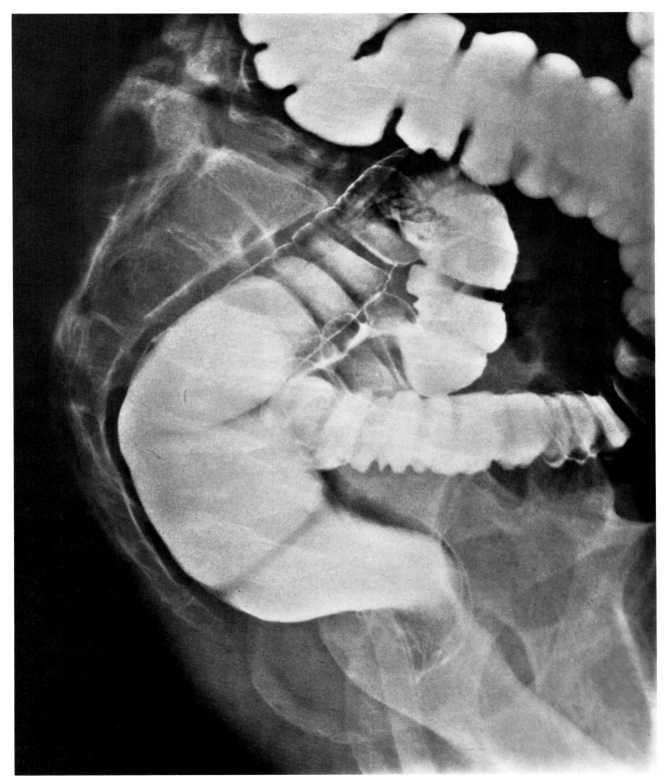

Fig. 140. Barium enema (rectum and sigmoid colon, lateral view)

Large Intestine

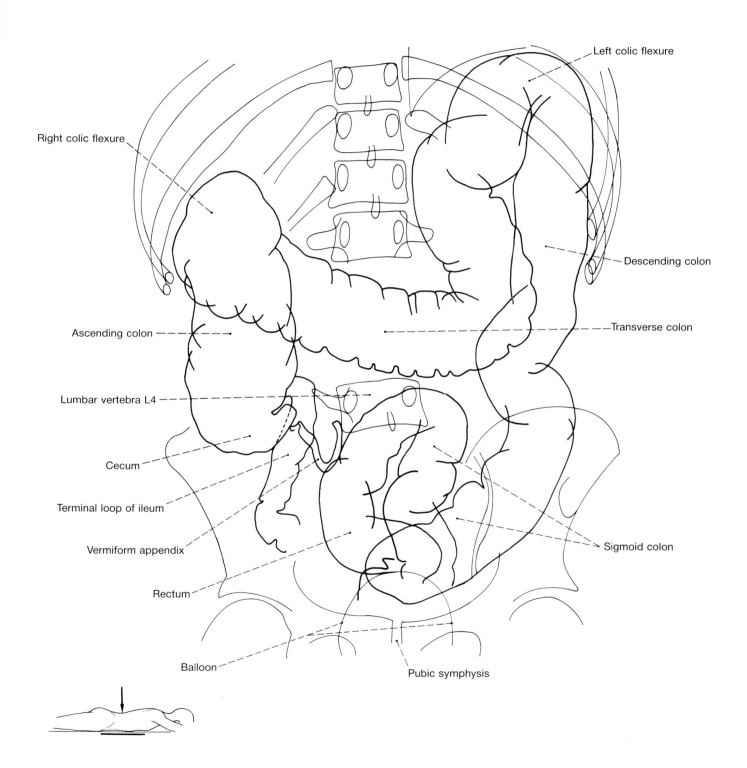

Left colic flexure

Right colic flexure

Descending colon

Ascending colon

Transverse colon

Lumbar vertebra L4

Cecum

Terminal loop of ileum

Vermiform appendix

Sigmoid colon

Rectum

Balloon

Pubic symphysis

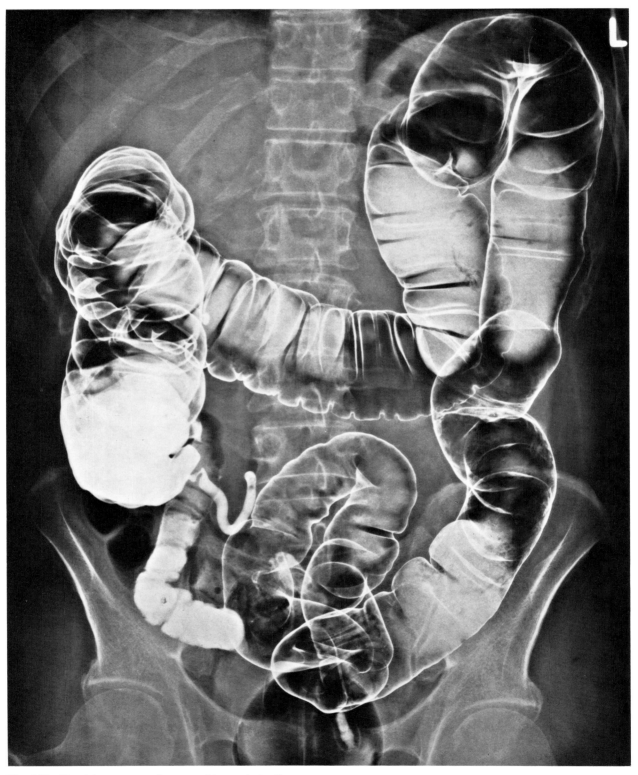

Fig. 141. Double-contrast image of large intestine

Gall Bladder and Biliary Ducts

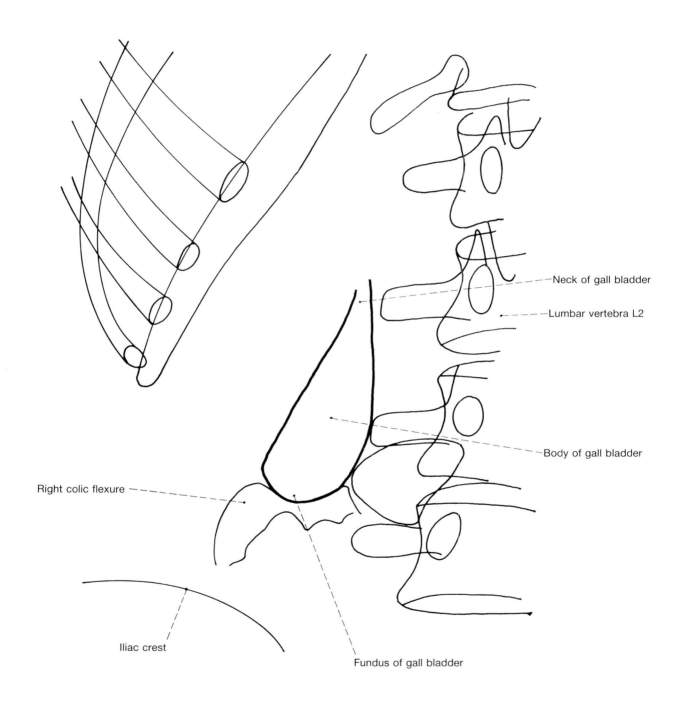

Neck of gall bladder

Lumbar vertebra L2

Body of gall bladder

Right colic flexure

Iliac crest

Fundus of gall bladder

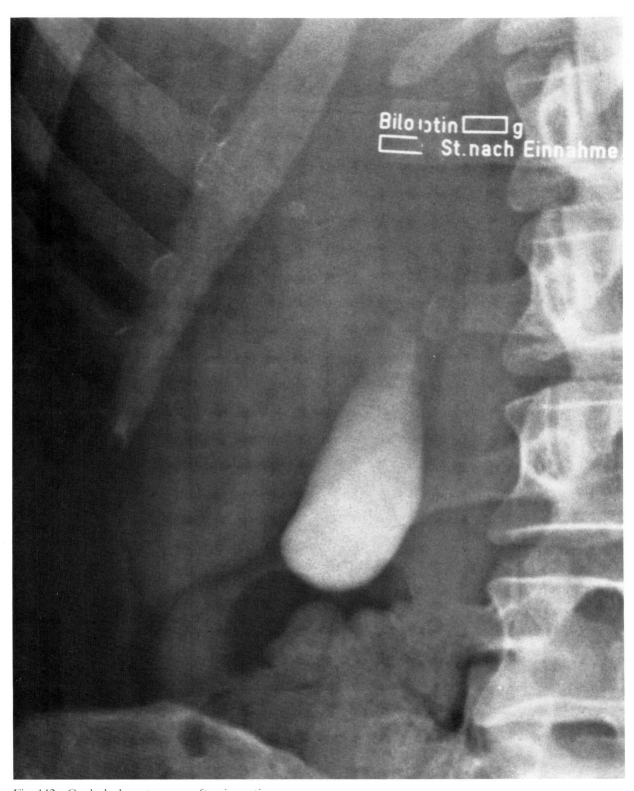

Fig. 142. Oral cholecystogram after ingestion

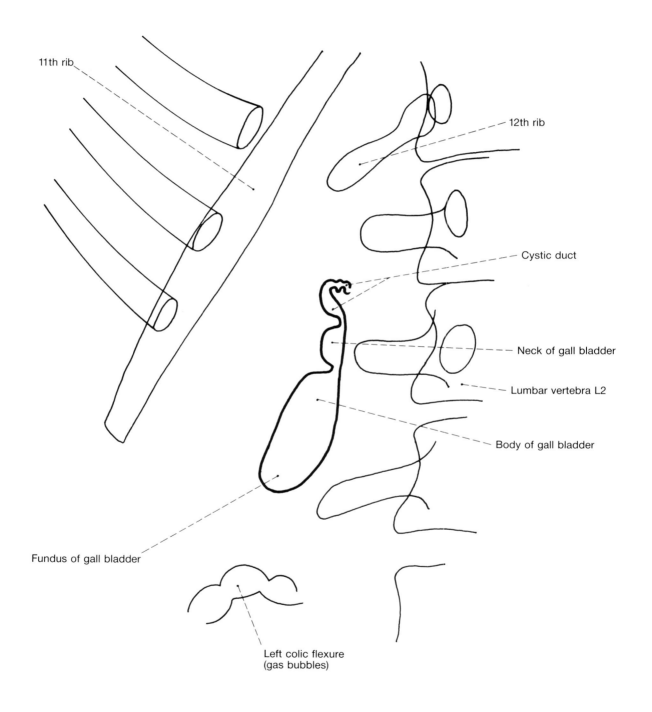

11th rib

12th rib

Cystic duct

Neck of gall bladder

Lumbar vertebra L2

Body of gall bladder

Fundus of gall bladder

Left colic flexure
(gas bubbles)

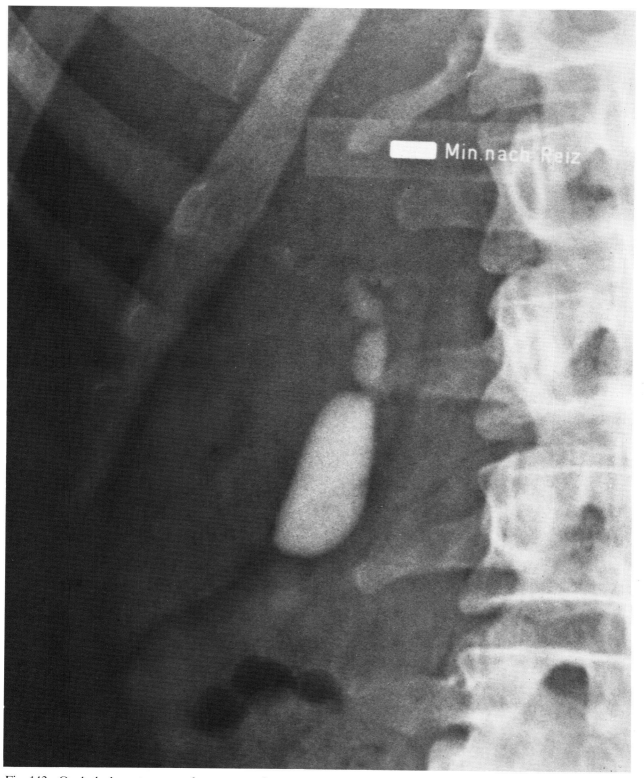

Min.nach Reiz

Fig. 143. Oral cholecystogram after contraction

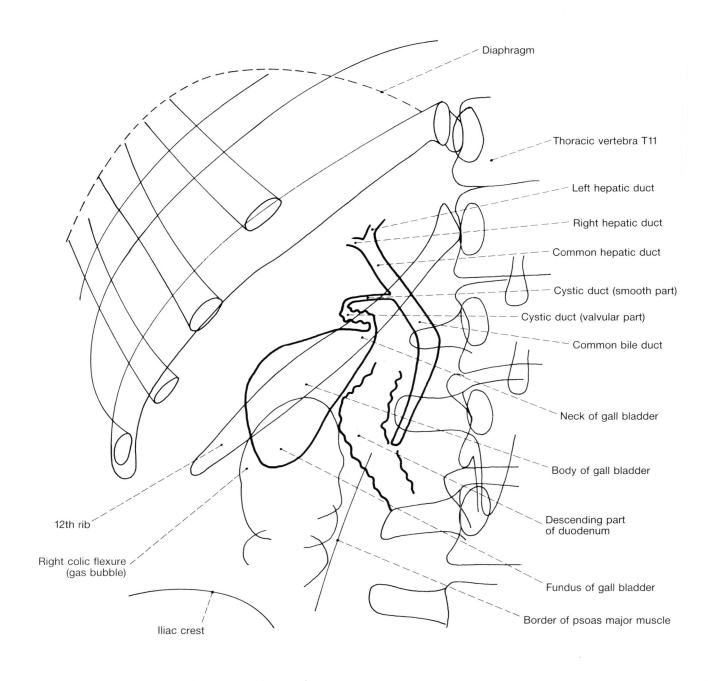

Diaphragm

Thoracic vertebra T11

Left hepatic duct

Right hepatic duct

Common hepatic duct

Cystic duct (smooth part)

Cystic duct (valvular part)

Common bile duct

Neck of gall bladder

Body of gall bladder

Descending part
of duodenum

Fundus of gall bladder

Border of psoas major muscle

12th rib

Right colic flexure
(gas bubble)

Iliac crest

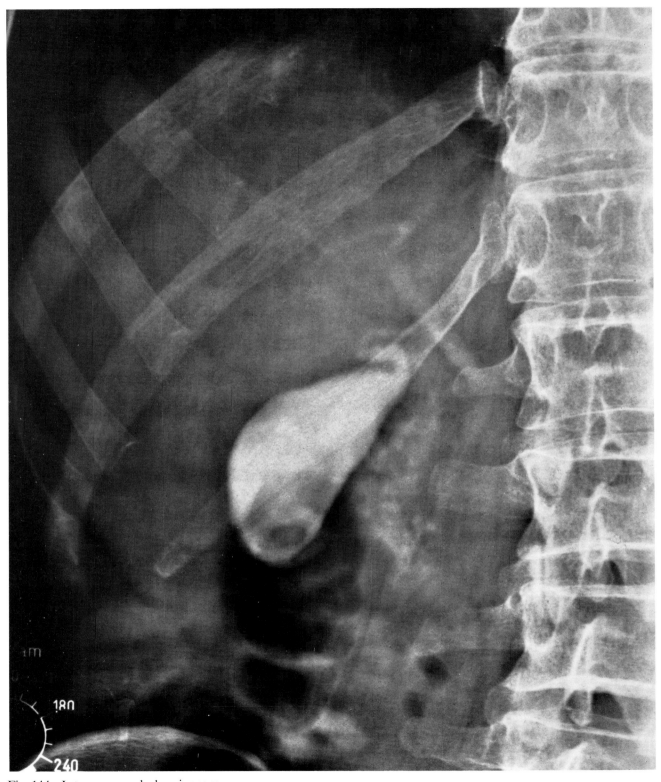

Fig. 144. Intravenous cholangiogram

Biliary Ducts, Cholangiography

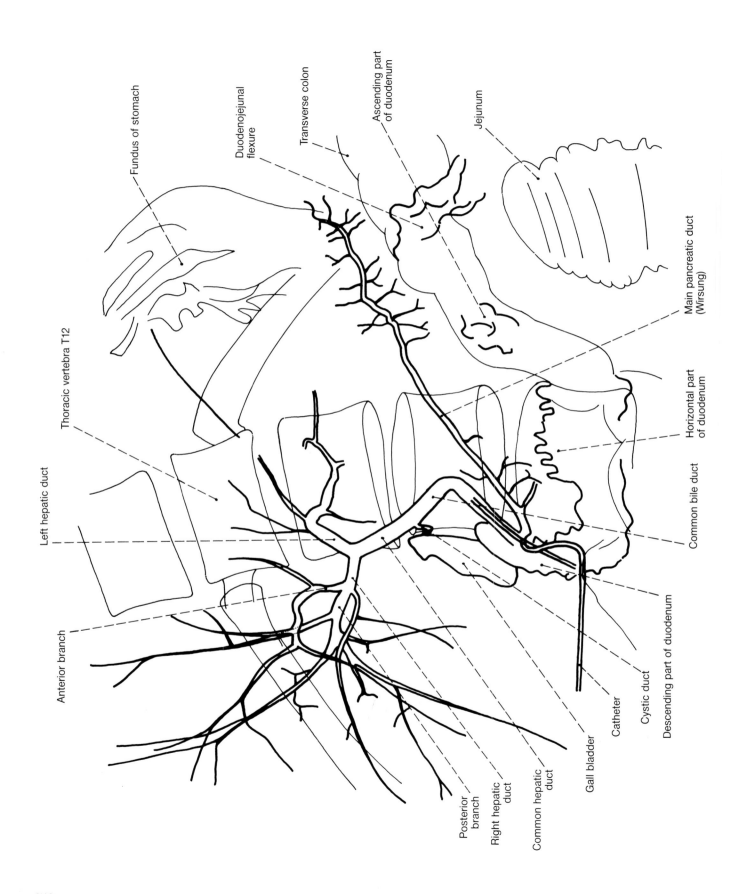

Fundus of stomach

Duodenojejunal flexure

Transverse colon

Ascending part of duodenum

Jejunum

Main pancreatic duct (Wirsung)

Thoracic vertebra T12

Horizontal part of duodenum

Left hepatic duct

Common bile duct

Anterior branch

Posterior branch

Right hepatic duct

Common hepatic duct

Gall bladder

Catheter

Cystic duct

Descending part of duodenum

242

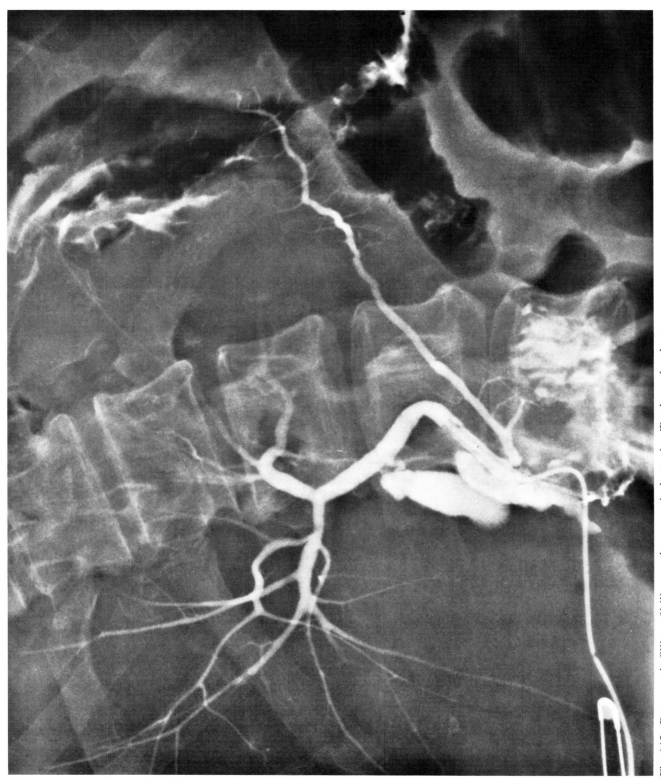

Fig. 145. Retrograde filling of biliary and pancreatic ducts via a T-tube and catheter

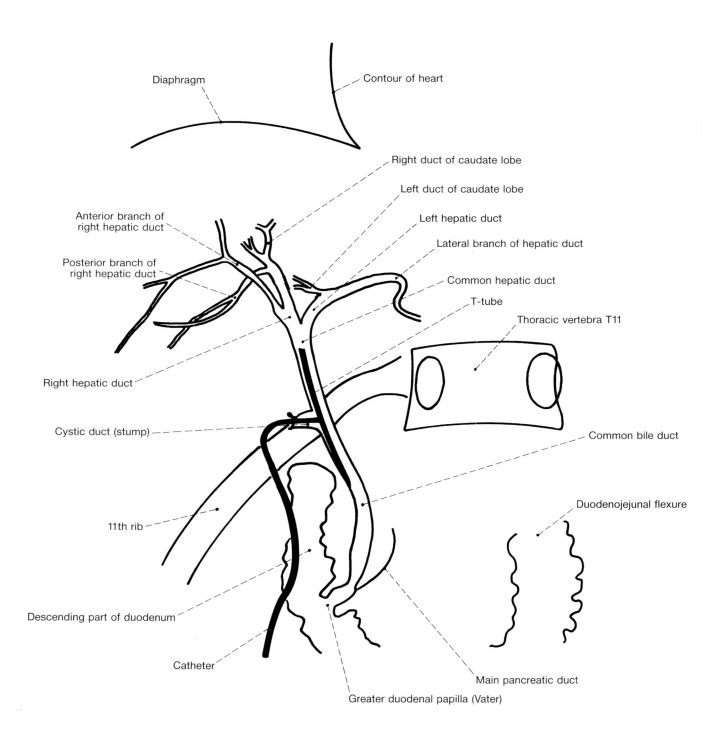

Diaphragm

Contour of heart

Right duct of caudate lobe

Left duct of caudate lobe

Anterior branch of
right hepatic duct

Left hepatic duct

Lateral branch of hepatic duct

Posterior branch of
right hepatic duct

Common hepatic duct

T-tube

Thoracic vertebra T11

Right hepatic duct

Cystic duct (stump)

Common bile duct

Duodenojejunal flexure

11th rib

Descending part of duodenum

Catheter

Main pancreatic duct

Greater duodenal papilla (Vater)

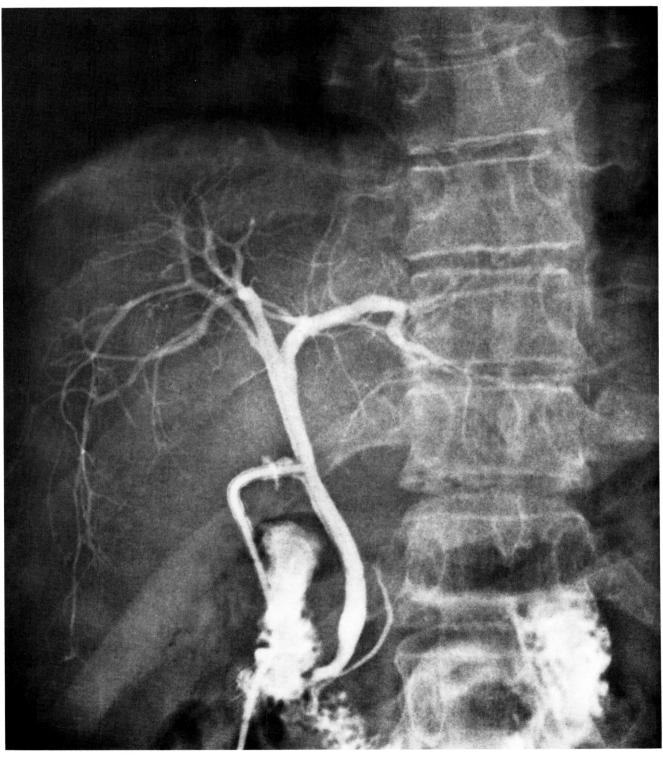

Fig. 146. Intraoperative cholangiogram of the biliary ducts

Kidneys and Urinary Tract

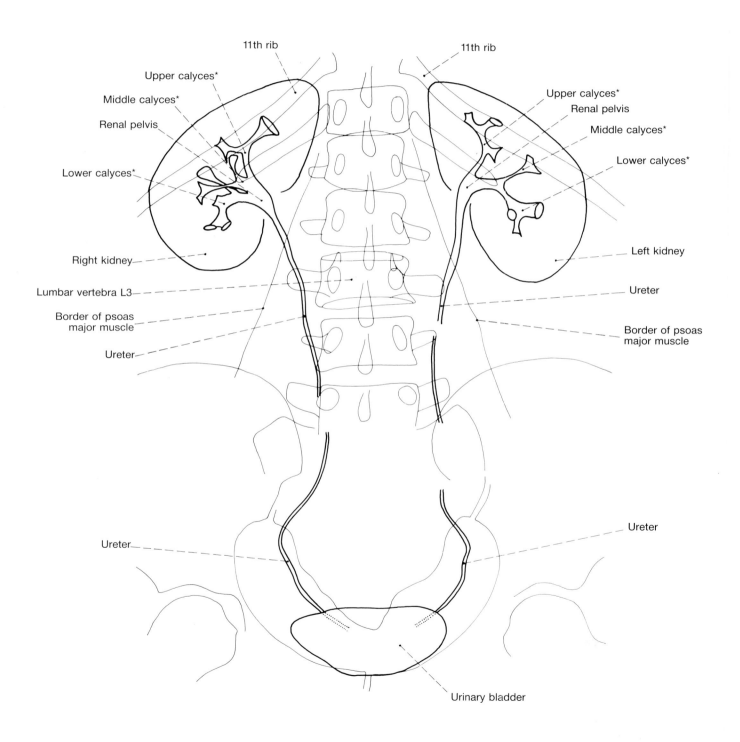

11th rib

11th rib

Upper calyces*

Upper calyces*

Renal pelvis

Middle calyces*

Middle calyces*

Renal pelvis

Lower calyces*

Lower calyces*

Lower calyces*

Right kidney

Left kidney

Lumbar vertebra L3

Ureter

Border of psoas major muscle

Border of psoas major muscle

Ureter

Ureter

Ureter

Urinary bladder

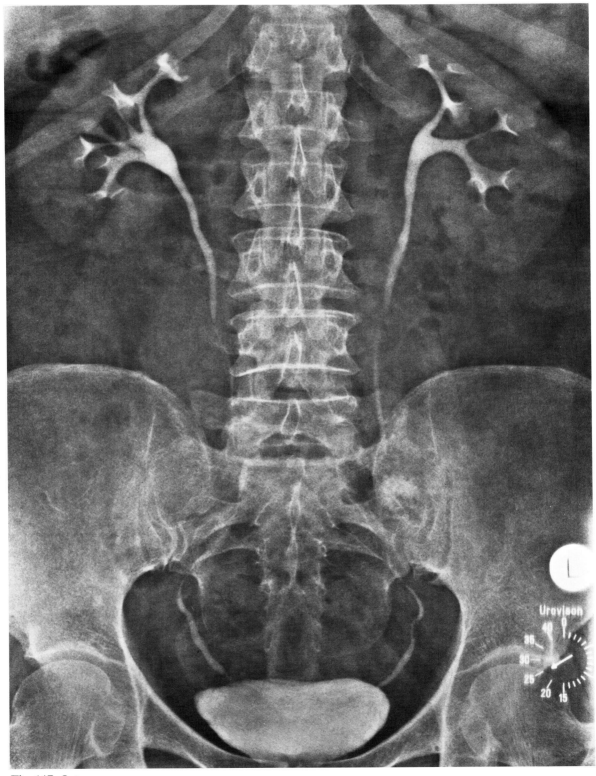

Fig. 147. Intravenous urogram

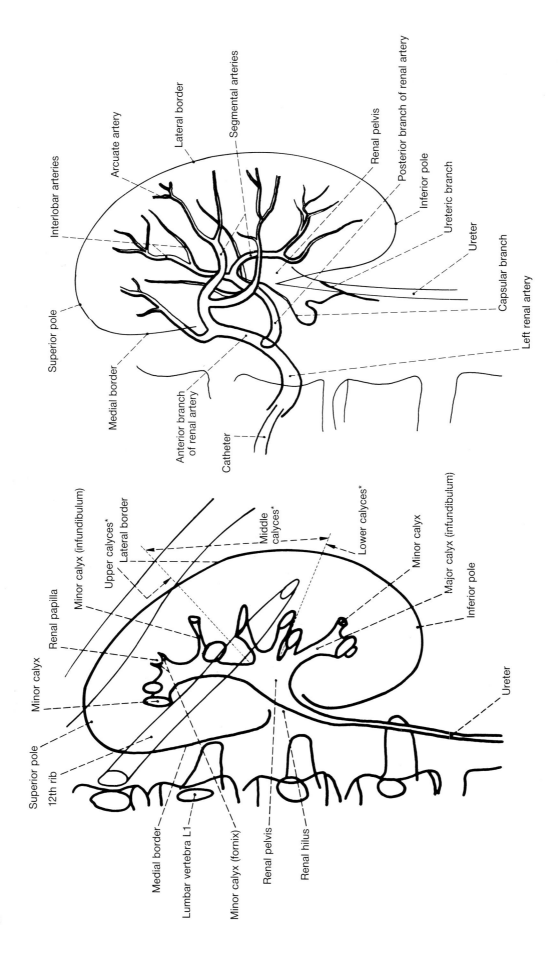

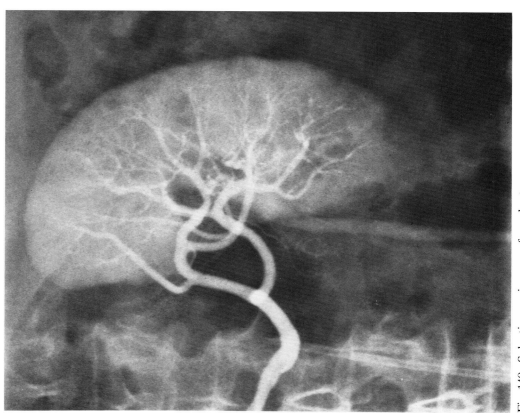

Fig. 149. Selective angiogram of renal artery

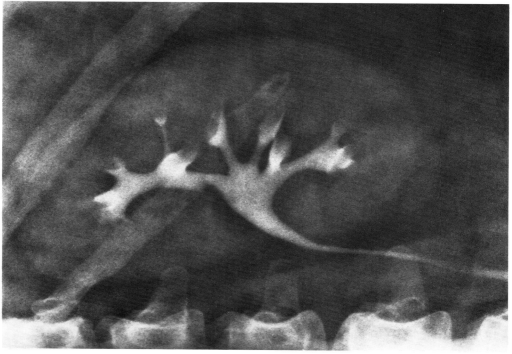

Fig. 148. Intravenous urogram (section of left kidney)

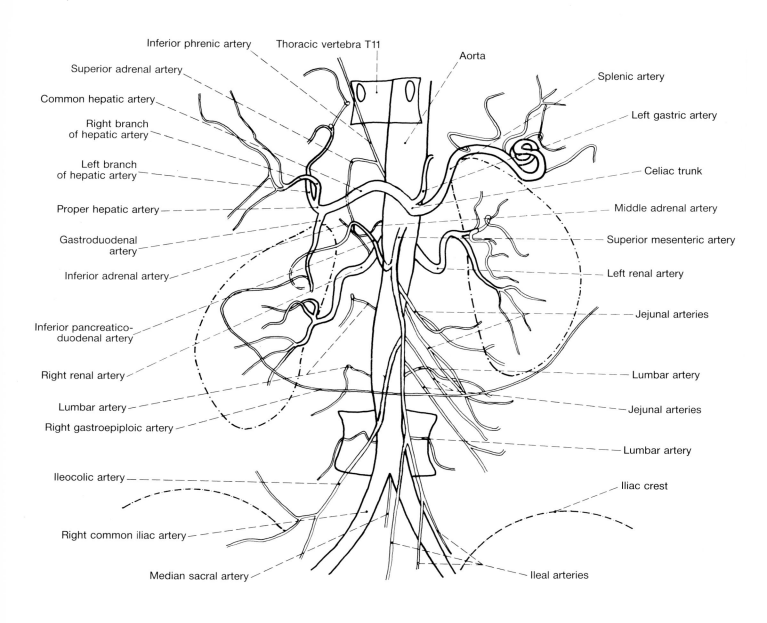

Inferior phrenic artery

Thoracic vertebra T11

Aorta

Superior adrenal artery

Common hepatic artery

Right branch
of hepatic artery

Left branch
of hepatic artery

Proper hepatic artery

Gastroduodenal
artery

Inferior adrenal artery

Inferior pancreatico-
duodenal artery

Right renal artery

Lumbar artery

Right gastroepiploic artery

Ileocolic artery

Right common iliac artery

Median sacral artery

Splenic artery

Left gastric artery

Celiac trunk

Middle adrenal artery

Superior mesenteric artery

Left renal artery

Jejunal arteries

Lumbar artery

Jejunal arteries

Lumbar artery

Iliac crest

Ileal arteries

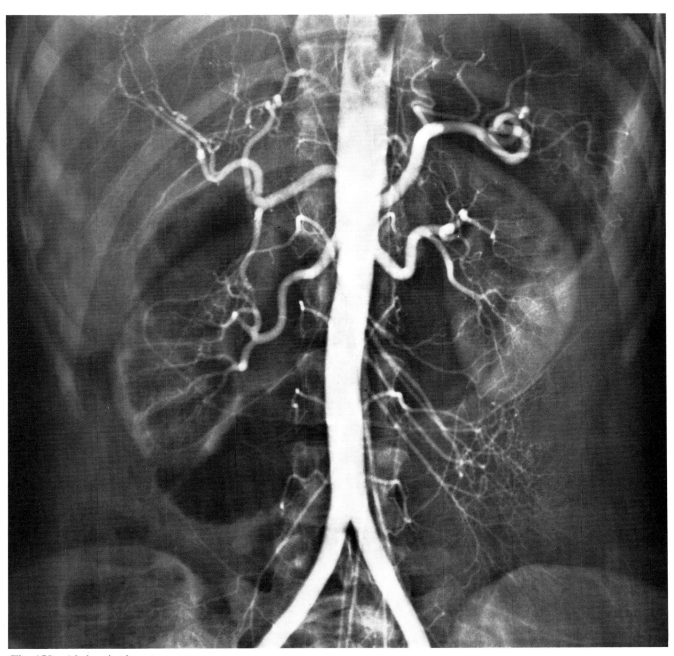

Fig. 150. Abdominal aortogram

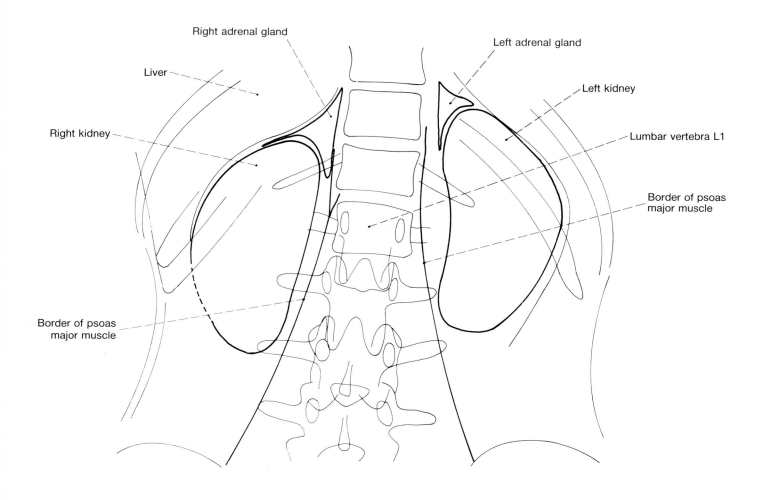

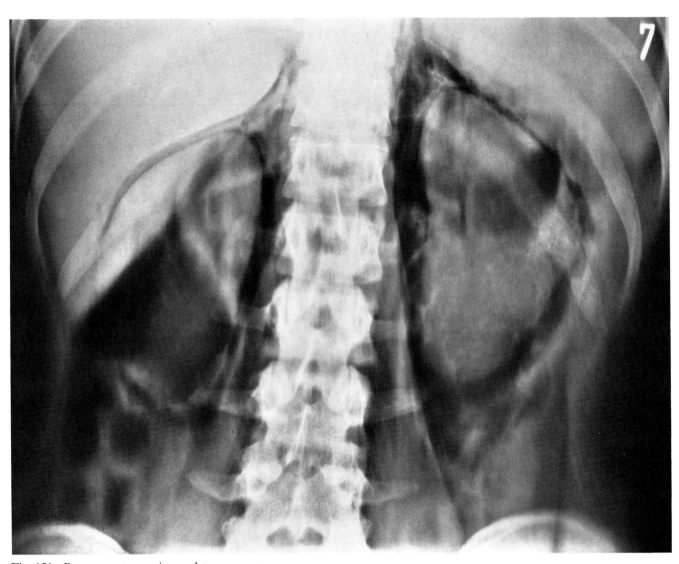

Fig. 151. Pneumoretroperitoneal tomogram

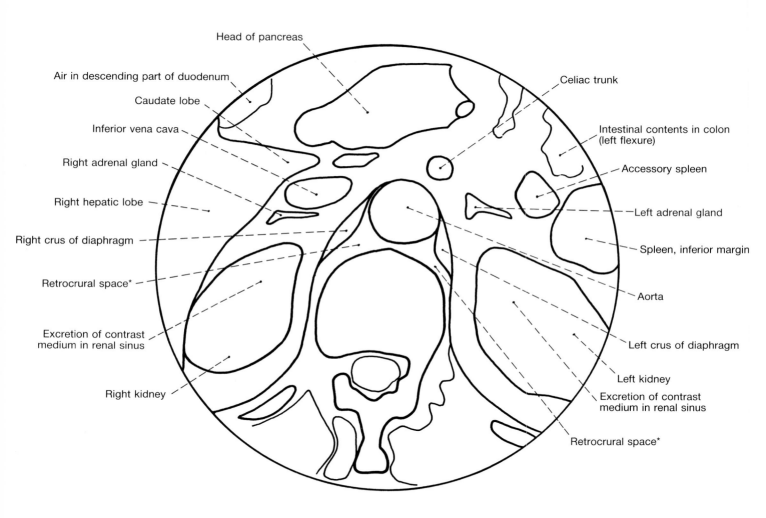

Head of pancreas

Air in descending part of duodenum

Caudate lobe

Inferior vena cava

Right adrenal gland

Right hepatic lobe

Right crus of diaphragm

Retrocrural space*

Excretion of contrast
medium in renal sinus

Right kidney

Celiac trunk

Intestinal contents in colon
(left flexure)

Accessory spleen

Left adrenal gland

Spleen, inferior margin

Aorta

Left crus of diaphragm

Left kidney

Excretion of contrast
medium in renal sinus

Retrocrural space*

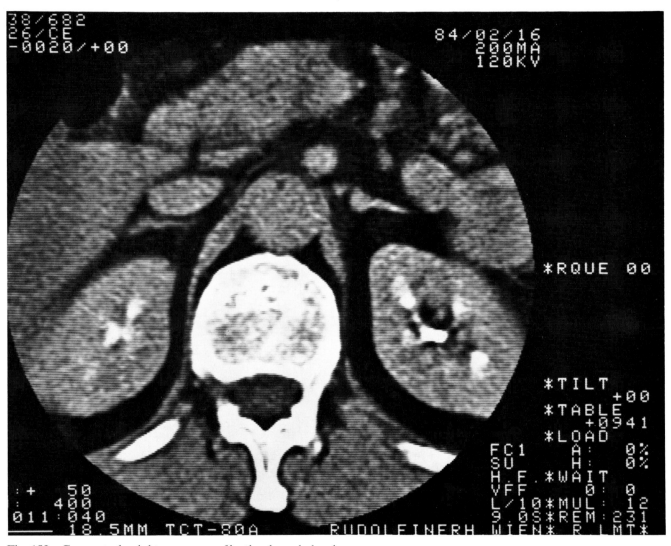

Fig. 152. Computed axial tomogram of both adrenal glands

Veins

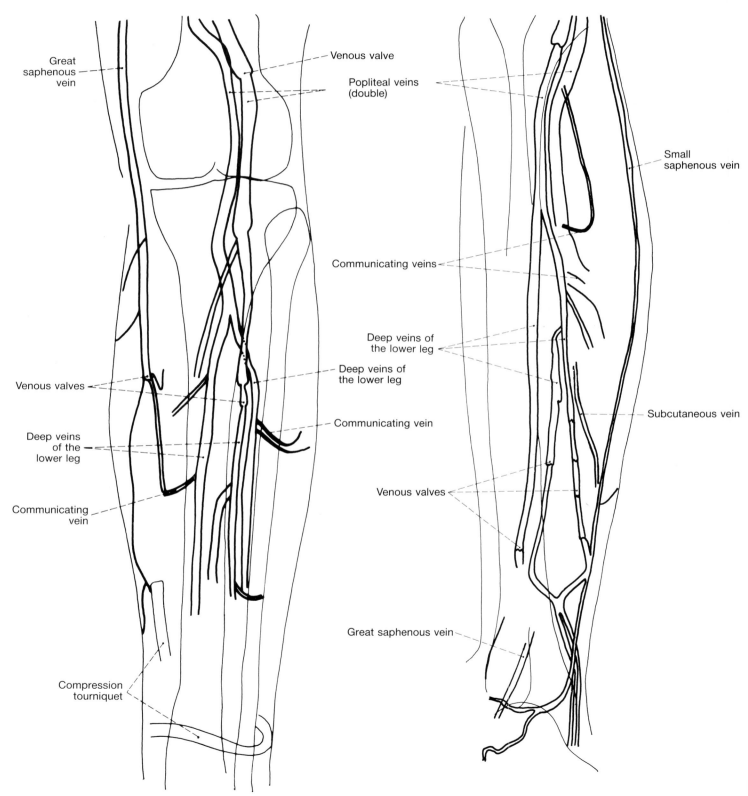

Great saphenous vein

Venous valve

Popliteal veins (double)

Small saphenous vein

Communicating veins

Deep veins of the lower leg

Deep veins of the lower leg

Venous valves

Communicating vein

Subcutaneous vein

Deep veins of the lower leg

Communicating vein

Venous valves

Great saphenous vein

Compression tourniquet

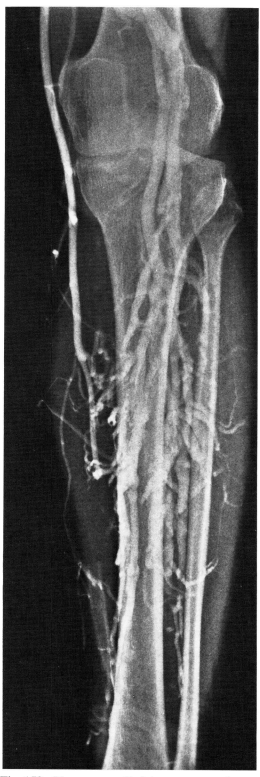

Fig. 153. Venogram of left lower extremity, a.p. view

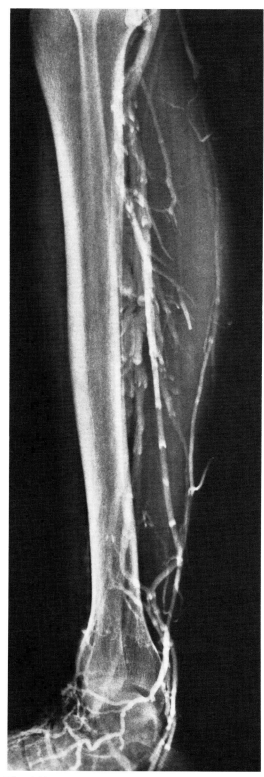

Fig. 154. Venogram of left lower extremity, lateral view

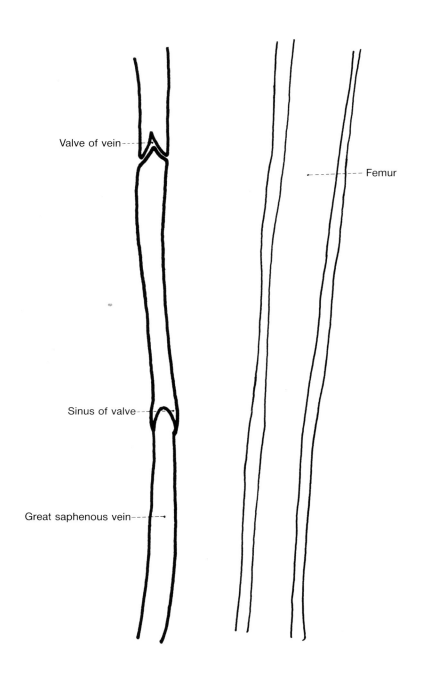

Valve of vein

Femur

Sinus of valve

Great saphenous vein

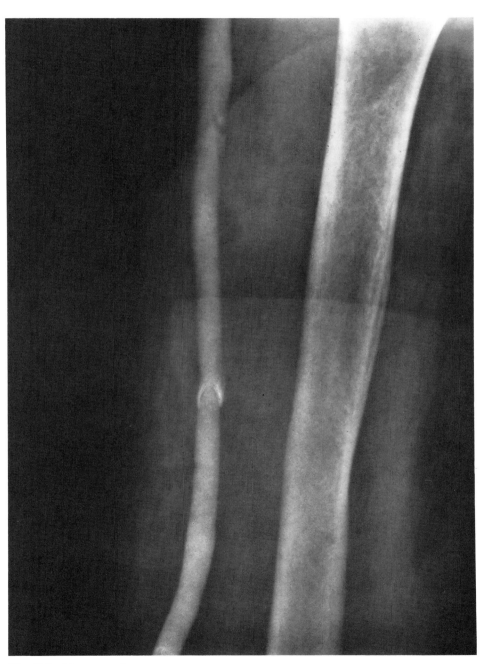

Fig. 155. Venous valve

Lymphatic System

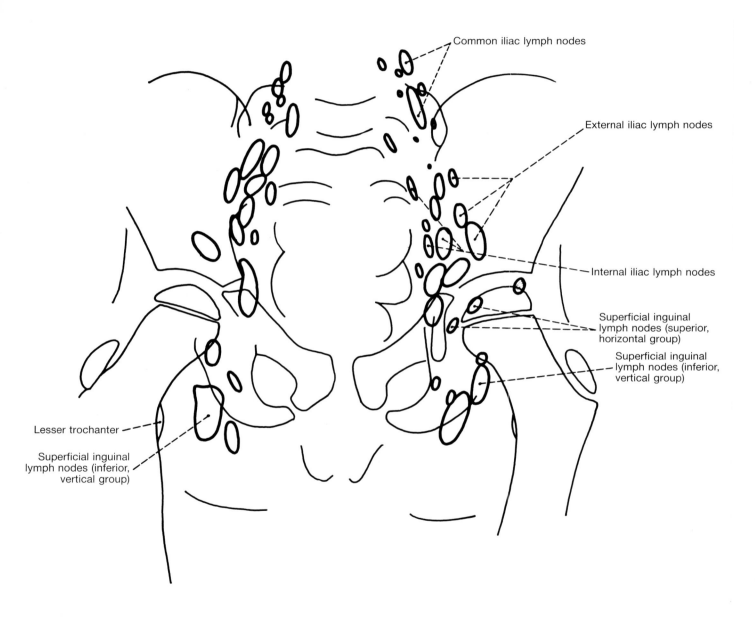

Common iliac lymph nodes

External iliac lymph nodes

Internal iliac lymph nodes

Superficial inguinal
lymph nodes (superior,
horizontal group)

Superficial inguinal
lymph nodes (inferior,
vertical group)

Lesser trochanter

Superficial inguinal
lymph nodes (inferior,
vertical group)

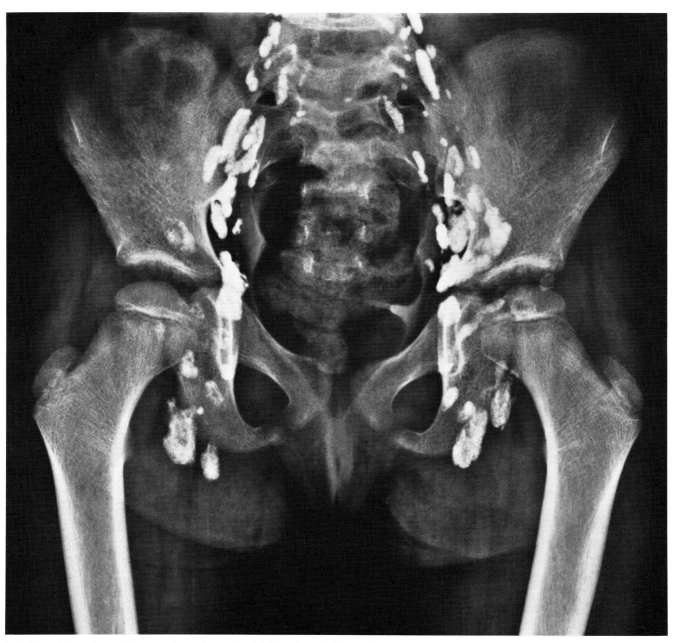

Fig. 156. Lymphangiogram of pelvic nodes (delayed study) a.p. view

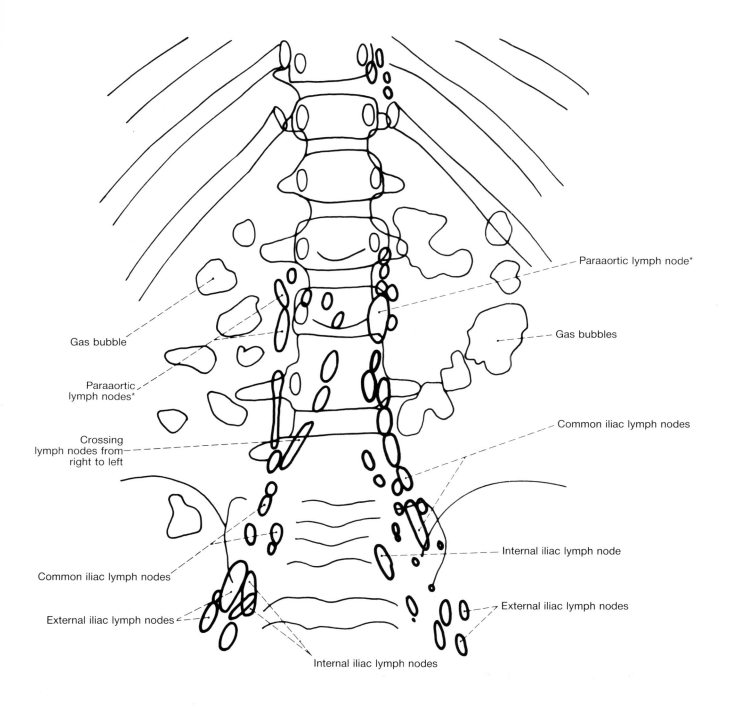

Paraaortic lymph node*

Gas bubble

Gas bubbles

Paraaortic
lymph nodes*

Common iliac lymph nodes

Crossing
lymph nodes from
right to left

Internal iliac lymph node

Common iliac lymph nodes

External iliac lymph nodes

External iliac lymph nodes

Internal iliac lymph nodes

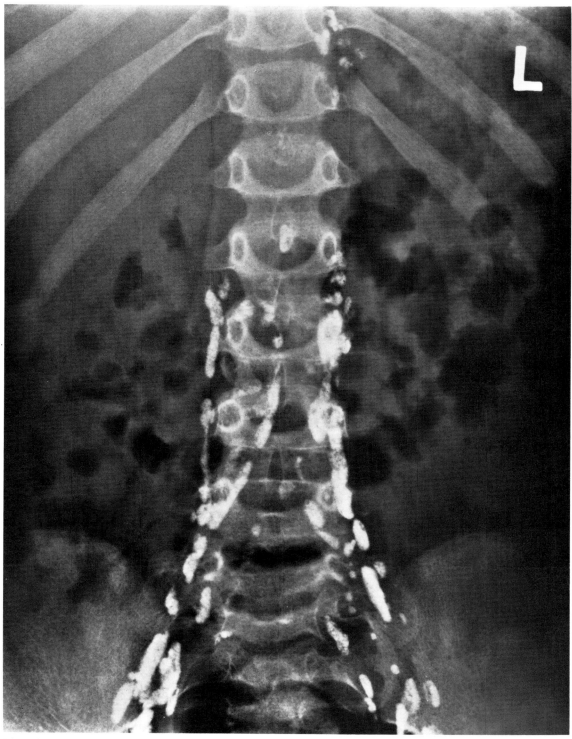

Fig. 157. Lymphangiogram of abdominal paraaortic nodes (delayed study), a.p. view

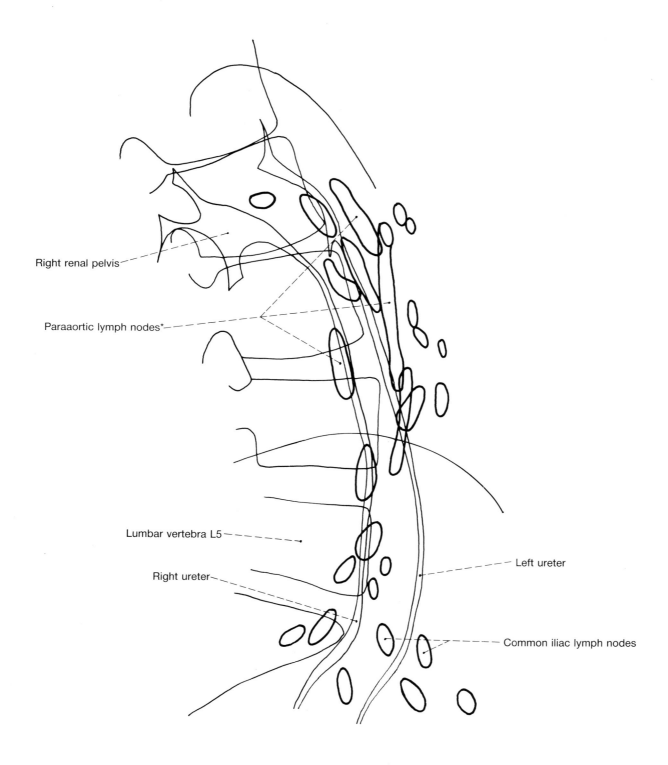

Right renal pelvis

Paraaortic lymph nodes*

Lumbar vertebra L5

Right ureter

Left ureter

Common iliac lymph nodes

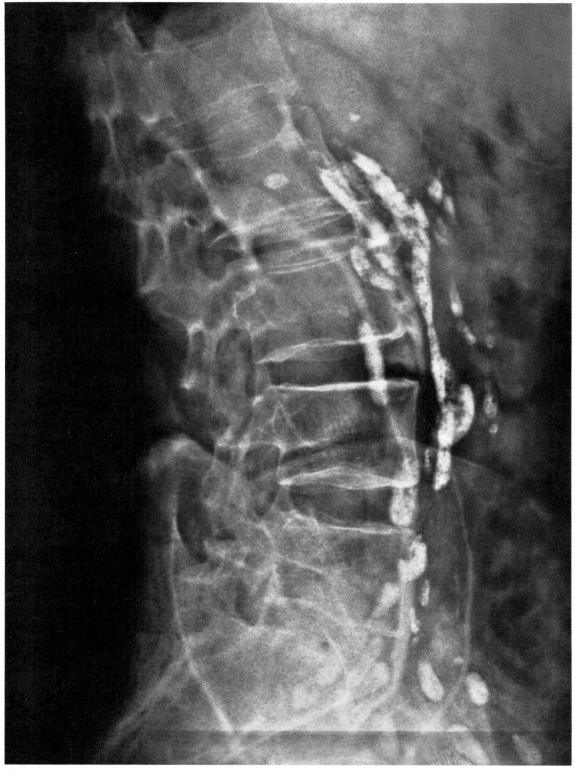

Fig. 158. Lymphangiogram of abdominal paraaortic nodes (delayed study), lateral view

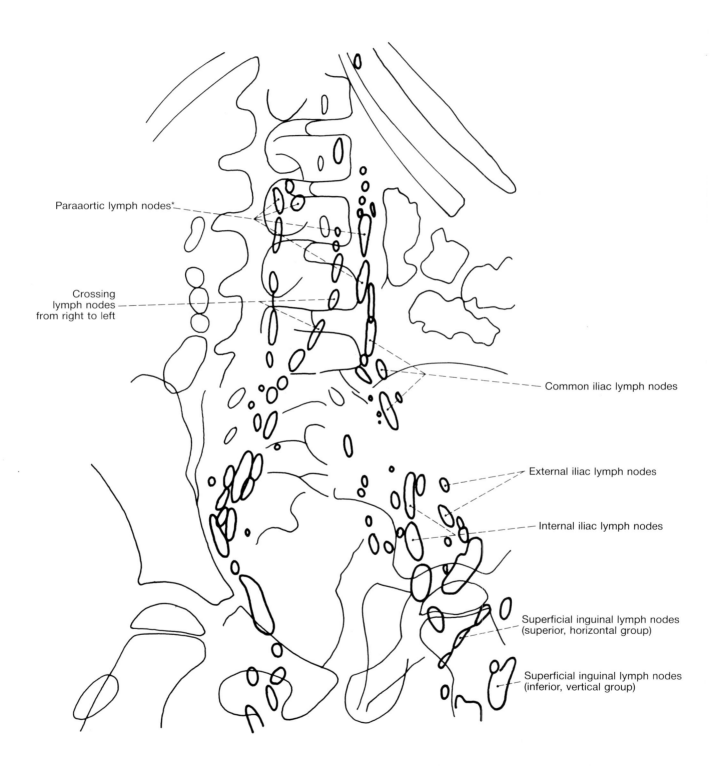

Paraaortic lymph nodes*

Crossing
lymph nodes
from right to left

Common iliac lymph nodes

External iliac lymph nodes

Internal iliac lymph nodes

Superficial inguinal lymph nodes
(superior, horizontal group)

Superficial inguinal lymph nodes
(inferior, vertical group)

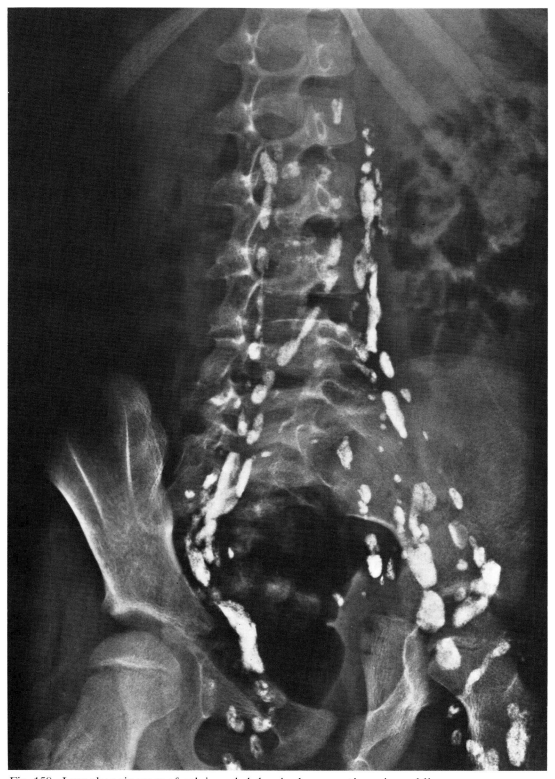

Fig. 159. Lymphangiogram of pelvic and abdominal paraaortic region, oblique

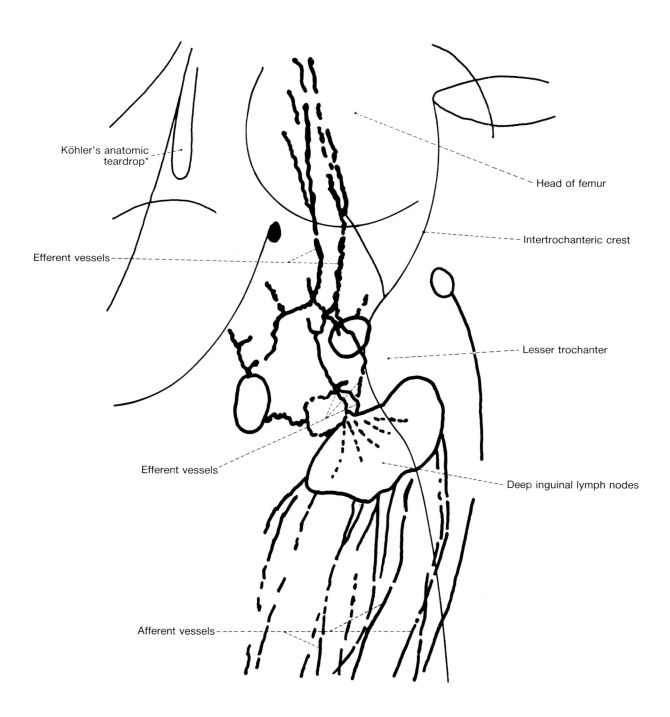

Köhler's anatomic teardrop*

Efferent vessels

Head of femur

Intertrochanteric crest

Lesser trochanter

Efferent vessels

Deep inguinal lymph nodes

Afferent vessels

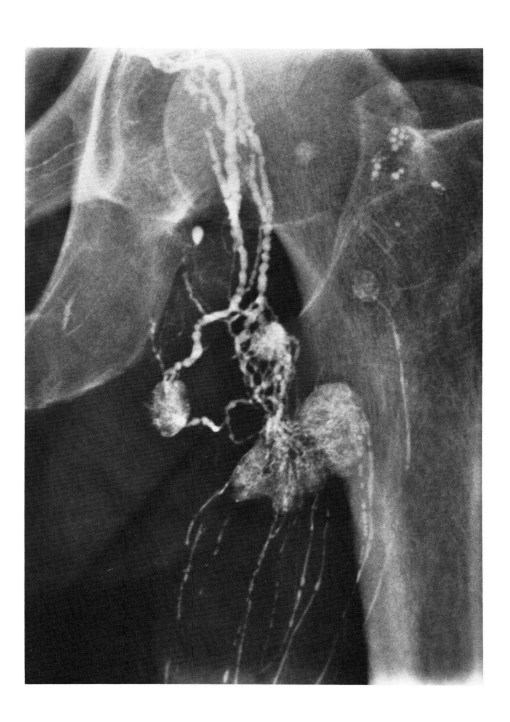

Fig. 160. Lymphangiogram
of inguinal lymph nodes
(filling phase)

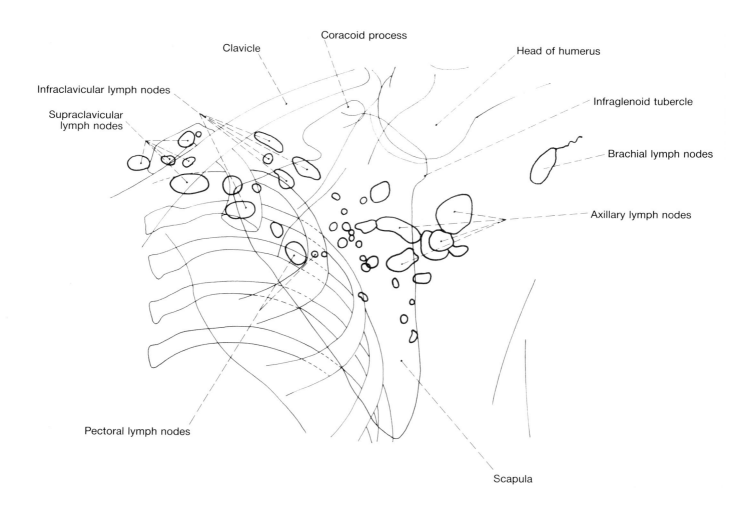

Coracoid process

Clavicle

Head of humerus

Infraclavicular lymph nodes

Infraglenoid tubercle

Supraclavicular
lymph nodes

Brachial lymph nodes

Axillary lymph nodes

Pectoral lymph nodes

Scapula

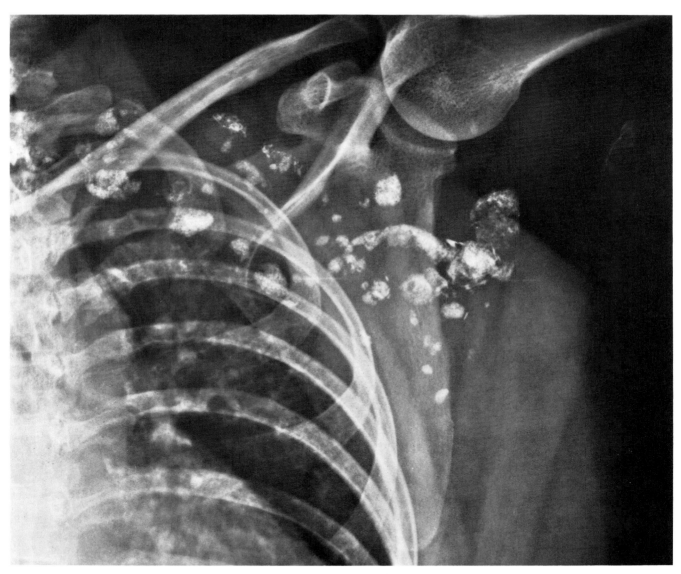

Fig. 161. Lymphangiogram of axillary lymph nodes (delayed study)

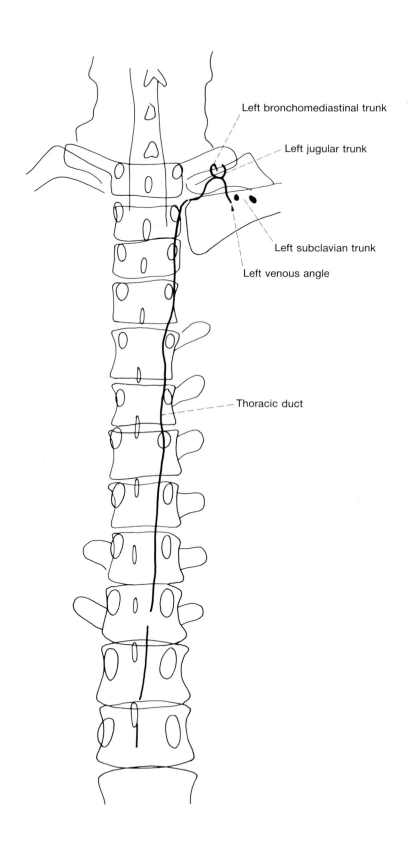

Left bronchomediastinal trunk

Left jugular trunk

Left subclavian trunk

Left venous angle

Thoracic duct

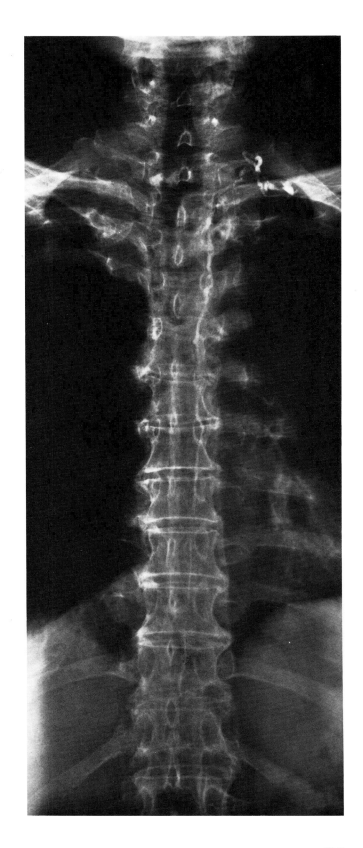

Fig. 162. Lymphangiogram of thoracic duct

Gynecologic Radiography

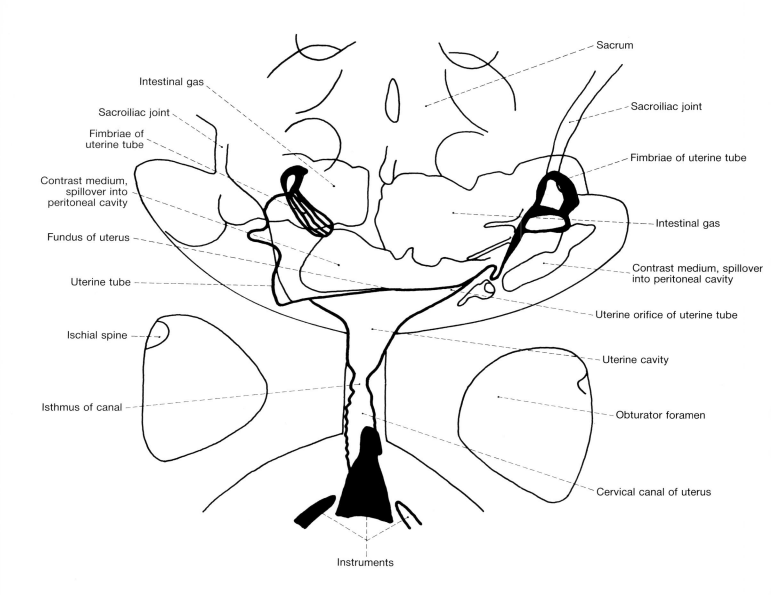

Intestinal gas

Sacroiliac joint

Fimbriae of
uterine tube

Contrast medium,
spillover into
peritoneal cavity

Fundus of uterus

Uterine tube

Ischial spine

Isthmus of canal

Sacrum

Sacroiliac joint

Fimbriae of uterine tube

Intestinal gas

Contrast medium, spillover
into peritoneal cavity

Uterine orifice of uterine tube

Uterine cavity

Obturator foramen

Cervical canal of uterus

Instruments

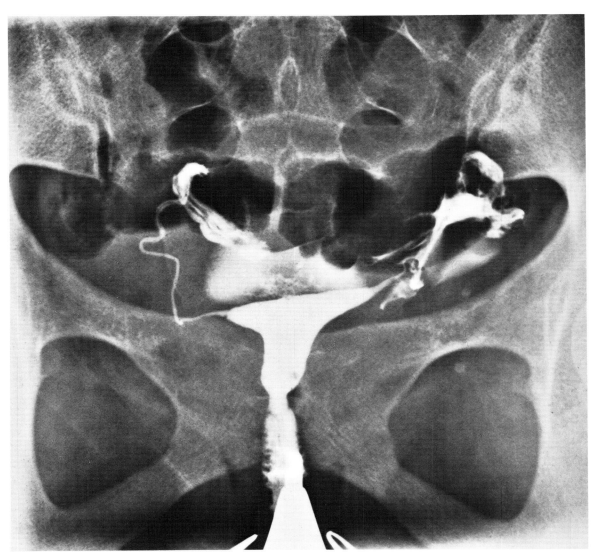

Fig. 163. Hysterosalpingogram

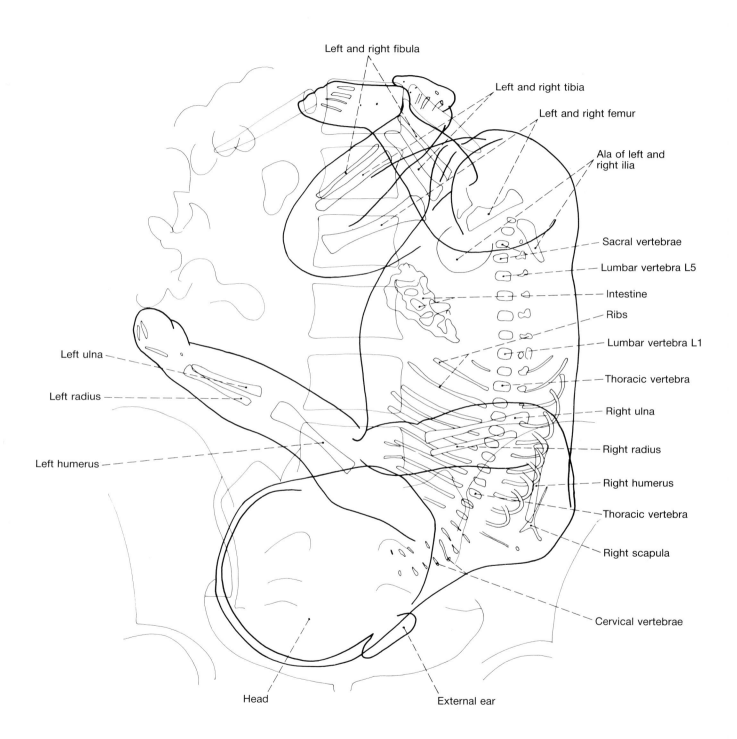

Left and right fibula

Left and right tibia

Left and right femur

Ala of left and
right ilia

Sacral vertebrae

Lumbar vertebra L5

Intestine

Ribs

Lumbar vertebra L1

Thoracic vertebra

Left ulna

Left radius

Right ulna

Right radius

Left humerus

Right humerus

Thoracic vertebra

Right scapula

Cervical vertebrae

Head

External ear

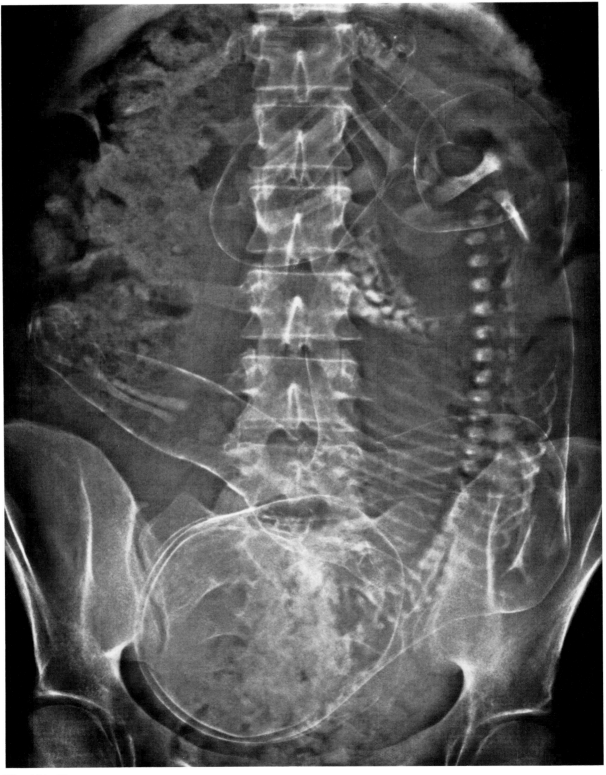

Fig. 164. Fetogram

Glossary

Anatomy: The science of the structure of the human body (from the Greek for dismember, dissect).

Angiocardiography: X-ray imaging of the cardiac chambers and great vessels after injection of a positive contrast medium through a catheterized leg or arm vein (direct method) or, infrequently, via injection into the veins of both arms simultaneously (peripheral angiocardiography).

Angiography: Radiologic method of imaging blood vessels by injection of contrast material into the arteries or veins of the vascular system.

Aortography: Radiographic imaging of the aorta and its large branches by injection of a positive contrast medium via catheterization or by percutaneous puncture.

Arteriography: Imaging of the arterial system of a given body region or of an organ system by means of a radiopaque contrast medium administered directly by injection or indirectly by catheterization.

Arthrography: Visualization of a joint by injection of a positive or, sometimes, a negative (double-contrast) contrast medium into the joint, thereby enabling the cartilaginous portions of the joint, the capsule interior, and the connecting bursae to be examined.

Bronchography: Radiographic examination of the inner surfaces of the trachea and bronchii by administration of a highly viscous positive contrast medium and air via an intratracheal tube, followed by inspiration.

Carotid angiography: Imaging of the carotid artery (mostly internal) and its branches by injection of a contrast material by either direct puncture or catheterization.

Cavography: Imaging of the superior and inferior vena cava.

Cerebral angiography: Examination of the vessels of the brain.

Cholangiography: Imaging of the large intra- and extrahepatic biliary ducts by intravenous injection of contrast medium that is extracted by the liver.

Cholecystangiography: Imaging of the gall bladder and biliary ducts by intravenous administration of contrast medium.

Cholecystography: Imaging of the gall bladder, either approximately 12 hours after oral administration of a radiopaque material (which is absorbed in the intestine and carried by the portal vein to the liver, where it is metabolized and excreted) or after intravenous injection.

Cisternography: Examination of the cerebral cisterns.

Compton effect: Exchange effect that occurs when x-rays impinge upon matter, whereby, after the electromagnetic radiation (photon) strikes, a portion of its energy is imparted to an electron in the form of oscillation energy and the photon departs with diminished energy (i. e., longer wavelength).

Computed tomography: Imaging method in which the x-ray tube rotates in various angular positions around the long axis of a body, transmitting data on the different absorption values of a given organ; from these data density maps are calculated and a cross-sectional picture is constructed, which is then recorded on magnetic tape and viewed on a screen.

Coronary angiography: Radiography of the coronary vessels by injection of a positive contrast material via selective catheterization of the right or left coronary artery.

Coronary arteriography: See coronary angiography.

Countercurrent angiography: Imaging of vessel sections above the injection site (toward the heart) by injecting contrast material at high pressure against the direction of blood flow.

Cystography: Examination of the gall bladder.
1. After intravenous administration (in conjunction with a urogram).
2. Retrograde, by injecting a radiopaque material via the urethra or a catheter in the urinary bladder, possibly using a double-contrast method.

Dacrycystography: Imaging of the lachrymal canal and duct.

Discography: Visualization of the intervertebral discs of the spine by injection of positive and negative contrast media into the nucleus pulposus.

Double-contrast imaging: Imaging of the inner surface of hollow organs by simultaneous use of positive and negative contrast media.

Encephalography: Imaging of the cerebral ventricles by using positive or negative contrast media (now mainly supplanted by computed tomography).

Fetography: Imaging of the surface of the fetus (or, rarely, its gastrointestinal tract) in the uterus after injection of a positive contrast medium into the amniotic sac.

Gastric radiography: Examination of the esophageal hiatus, stomach, and duodenum up to the duodenojejunal flexure with a barium sulfate suspension (in rare cases water-soluble Gastrografin) as a monocontrast method and supplemented with a negative contrast medium (air or gas) as a double-contrast method.

Hypotonic duodenography: Imaging of the duodenum by a double-contrast method after relaxation of the smooth muscles of the intestinal wall (e. g., with glucagon).

Hysterophlebography: Imaging of the veins of the uterus by injection of a contrast medium into the wall of the uterus from the uterine cavity.

Hysterosalpingography: Roentgenography of the uterus and oviducts.

Infusion cholecystangiography: Imaging of the gall bladder and ducts by slow infusion of a large amount of contrast material, as in cholecystangiography.

Infusion urography: Imaging of the kidneys, calyces of the renal pelvis, ureters, and urinary bladder by infusion of a larger quantity of diluted contrast material than used in urography.

Lactography: Imaging of the mammary duct of the female breast by using a positive contrast medium.

Lymphography: Radiography of the lymphatics (lymphangiography) and lymph nodes (lymphadenography) after injection of a radiopaque (iodinated, oily) contrast medium (Ethiodol) via a lymphatic made visible by a dye.

Magnetic resonance imaging (MRI): Formerly nuclear magnetic resonance (NMR). See nuclear spin tomography.

Mammography: Radiography of the female breast (in men, in rare cases) by using a special x-ray tube and film.

Mediastinography: See pneumomediastinography.

Mesenteric angiography: Radiographic examination of the superior or inferior mesenteric artery by injecting a contrast material via a catheterized vessel.

Micturition urethrography: Examination of the urethra during urination after previous filling of the urinary bladder.

Glossary

Myelography: Radiography of the subarachnoid spaces after direct injection of an oily (Pantopaque) or aqueous (Amipaque) iodinated contrast material into the spinal canal.

Nephrography: Examination of the kidneys (parenchyma) by means of urography or angiography.

Nuclear spin tomography: A diagnostic imaging method in which the axes of hydrogen atoms, for example, within human tissue (soft tissue diagnosis) placed within the field of a large circular magnet (0.1 to 2.0 tesla) are aligned in parallel and then stimulated by high-frequency radio waves. The resonant energy emitted by the excited nuclei when the high-frequency signal is removed is transmitted to a computer and calculated on a gray scale. The data are then arranged spatially so that the region under investigation can be viewed three-dimensionally.

Pancreatic radiography: Imaging of the pancreas after injection of a positive contrast material via a catheter inserted gastroscopically into the greater duodenal papilla of Vater.

Peripheral angiography: Radiography of the blood vessels of the upper or lower extremities after a direct injection of a positive contrast material (e.g., Renografin).

Pharmacoangiography: Examination of vessels or organs after injection of a pharmacologically active material into the vessels through an angiographic catheter, which is then followed by injection of a contrast material.

Pharmacoradiography: Radiologic method combined with pharmacologic challenge of various organ systems.

Phlebography: See venography.

Photoelectric effect: Exchange effect occurring when high-energy electromagnetic radiation strikes material.

Planography: See tomography.

Pneumoarthrography: Radiography of the joint cavities that uses a negative contrast material.

Pneumocystography: Radiography of the bladder that uses a negative contrast material.

Pneumoencephalography: Radiography of the cerebral ventricles that uses a negative contrast medium (now almost entirely superceded by computed tomography).

Pneumomediastinography: Radiography of the mediastinum that uses a negative contrast material.

Pneumoretroperitonography: Radiography of the retroperitoneal organs after injection of negative contrast material into the connective tissue in front of the sacrum.

Pulmonary angiography: Examination of the pulmonary artery and its branches by injection of a contrast medium via a catheter inserted into a vein of the arm or leg.

Pyelography: Radiography of the kidney, pelvic calyces, ureters, and bladder using a radiopaque material (e.g., Conray).
1. Intravenous pyelography (abbreviated IVP): Performed after intravenously administered positive contrast medium is excreted by the kidneys. (A more appropriate designation would be excretory pyelography or urography.)
2. Retrograde pyelography: Examination of the pelvic calyces of the kidney by injecting a positive contrast material into a catheter inserted into the ureter as far as the renal pelvis.

Renal angiography: Radiography of the renal vessels during exploratory angiography of the abdominal aorta or in selective angiography after catheterization.

Renovasography: See renal angiography.

Retrograde pyelography: See pyelography.

Selective angiography: Radiography of large arterial or venous vessels by injection of a positive contrast material via a catheter or directly (rare).

Sialography: Examination of the salivary glands by injection of a positive contrast material into the ducts.

Sinography: Imaging of a sinus tract by injection of a positive contrast medium into the sinus or canal.

Splenoportography: Examination of the splenic vein and the portal vein.
1. Direct splenoportography: After direct puncture of the spleen, a contrast material is injected into the puncture cannula and the efferent venous system is delineated.
2. Indirect splenoportography: Delineation of the splenic and portal veins in connection with celiac or possibly simultaneous mesenteric radiography.

Stray radiation raster: A laminated lead grid (moving or fixed) designed to eliminate scattered radiation.

Superselective angiography: Selective imaging of peripheral sections or branches of major arteries (for example, angiography of the gastroduodenal artery).

Thoracic aortography: Contrast medium delineation of the thoracic aorta.

Tomography: Sectional radiography producing sharp depiction of a specific body section while the overlying and underlying sections are blurred. Forms: linear, circular, elliptical, hypocycloidal, spiral.

Upper gastrointestinal series: Follow-through examination of the esophagus, stomach, and duodenum by means of a barium sulfate suspension and observation of the rate of barium passage (2 hours postconsumption).

Urethrography: Examination of the urethra by using a radiopaque material either via retrograde injection or via micturition urethrography.

Urography: Examination of the kidneys, renal pelvic calyces, ureter, and bladder after administration of contrast material taken up by the kidneys.

Venography: Examination of veins in a given region via direct puncture and injection into a superficial vein or, rarely, through bone.

Ventriculography: Radiography of the cerebral ventricles using a positive or negative contrast medium.

Vesiculography: Examination of the seminal vesicles after injection of a radiopaque material into the vas deferens.

Zonography: Imaging method based on a principle similar to tomography, except that a smaller section angle is used and therefore a thicker section of the body can be examined.

Bibliography

Angerstein, W.: Lexikon der radiologischen Technik in der Medizin. 2. Aufl. VEB Thieme, Leipzig 1975.

Benninghoff-Goerttler: Lehrbuch der Anatomie des Menschen Bd. 1, 12. Aufl. 1978; Bd. 2, 12. Aufl. 1979; Bd. 3, 11./12. Aufl. 1979. Urban & Schwarzenberg, München–Berlin–Wien.

Birkner, R.: Das typische Röntgenbild des Skelettes. Urban & Schwarzenberg, München–Berlin 1977.

Bontrager, K. L., B. T. Anthony: Textbook of Radiographic Positioning and Related Anatomy. Multi-Media Publishing, Inc., Denver, Colorado 1982.

Bunde, E.: Medizinische Röntgentechnik. Thieme, Stuttgart 1958. DIN 6814: Begriffe und Benennungen in der radiologischen Technik.

Ewen, K., G. Schmitt: Grundlagen des praktischen Strahlenschutzes an medizinischen Röntgeneinrichtungen. Enke, Stuttgart 1975.

Frik, W., U. Goering: Röntgenanatomie. 2. Aufl. Thieme, Stuttgart 1975.

Frommhold, W., H. Gajewski, H. D. Schoen: Medizinische Röntgentechnik. Bd. 1: Physikalische und technische Grundlagen, 4. Aufl. 1979. Bd. 2: Skelettaufnahmen, in Vorbereitung. Thieme, Stuttgart.

Goldhamer, K.: Normale Anatomie des Kopfes im Röntgenbild. In: Radiologische Praktika Bd. XII (1930), Bd. XIII (1931). Thieme, Leipzig.

Janker, K.: Röntgenbilder. Atlas der normierten Aufnahmen. Röntgenaufnahmetechnik II. 9. Aufl. Springer, Berlin–Heidelberg–New York 1976.

Kretschmann, H.-J., M. Kaltenbach: Anatomy and Nomenclature of Coronary Arteries. Coronary Heart Disease. International Symposium in Frankfurt. 22.–24. 1. 1970. Thieme, Stuttgart 1971.

Lippert, H., H. P. Lehamn: SI Units in Medicine, Urban & Schwarzenberg, Baltimore–Munich 1978.

May, R., R. Nißl: Die Phlebographie der unteren Extremität. 2. Aufl. Thieme, Stuttgart 1973.

Mayer, E. G.: Diagnose und Differentialdiagnose in der Schädelröntgenologie. Springer, Wien 1959.

Meschan, I.: An Atlas of Anatomy Basic to Radiology. W. B. Saunders Company, Philadelphia–London–Toronto 1975.

Nomina Anatomica, 4th edition. Excerpta Medica, Amsterdam–Oxford 1977.

Sauter, F.: Grundlagen des Strahlenschutzes. Siemens AG (1971).

Scherer, E.: Strahlentherapie. 2. Aufl. Thieme, Stuttgart 1973.

Schlungbaum, W.: Medizinische Strahlenkunde. 6. Aufl. De Gruyter, Berlin 1979.

Seeram, E.: X-Ray Imaging Equipment, an Introduction. Charles C. Thomas, Springfield, Illinois 1985.

Simon, G., W. J. Hamilton: X-Ray Anatomy. Butterworth, London 1978.

Simon, G.: Principles of Chest X-Ray Diagnosis. 4th Ed. Butterworth, London 1978.

Toldt-Hochstetter: Anatomischer Atlas, Bd. 1, 27. Aufl. 1979; Bd. 2, 27. Aufl. 1979. Urban & Schwarzenberg, München–Berlin–Wien.

Wenz, W.: Abdominale Angiographie. Springer, Berlin–Heidelberg–New York 1972.

Wicke, L., W. Firbas: Beitrag über die arterielle Gefäßversorgung des Herzens, Herz/Kreislauf 7, Nr. 5 (1975) 256–262.

Winau, R.: Wilhelm Conrad Röntgen. 1845–1923. Moos-Verlag, München 1973.

Zdansky, F.: Röntgendiagnostik des Herzens und der großen Gefäße. 3. Aufl. Springer, Wien 1962.

Zimmer, E. A., M. Brossy: Lehrbuch der röntgendiagnostischen Technik für Röntgenass. und Ärzte. 2. Aufl. Springer, Berlin–Heidelberg–New York 1974.

Subject Index

Abdomen, upper 228, 230
Acetabulum
– crest of 124
– fossa of 102, 124, 126, 128
– labrum of 102
– lunate surface of 102, 124, 126
– roof of 128
Acromion 108, 110
Ala
– of ilium 102
– fetal 276
– *see also* Wing
Alar folds 134
Ampulla, of rectum 232
Angle
– cardiovascular 166
– mandibular 2, 4, 62, 68, 70, 72, 196
– petrous (Angulus Citelli) 22
– of scapula
– – inferior 108
– – superior 62, 108, 150, 196
– of sternum 152, 186
– venous 172, 272
Angulus Citelli 22
Antrum, pyloric 208, 210, 212, 216
Aorta 78, 224, 228, 230, 250, 254
– abdominal 96, 106, 178
– arch (knob) of 150, 154, 166, 170,
   174, 176, 178, 180, 182, 204, 206
– ascending 168, 170, 174, 176, 178, 180,
   182
– bulb of 174
– descending 154, 166, 168, 170, 174, 176,
   180
– sinus of (Valsalva) 176, 190
– thoracic 82, 178, 182
– valve of 180
Apex
– of head of fibula 130, 132
– of petrous portion of temporal bone 22
– of pyramid 22
Appendix, vermiform 226, 234
Aqueduct, cerebral 50, 60
Arbor vitae 60. *See also* Vermis
Arch
– of aorta 150, 154, 166, 170, 174, 176,
   178, 180, 182, 204, 206
– of atlas 2, 4, 6, 64, 68, 202
– of cricoid cartilage 198
– dental
– – inferior 16, 18, 64
– – superior 16, 18, 64
– palmar arterial
– – deep 122
– – superficial 122

Arch, palmar
– pancreatic 220
– vertebral
– – lamina of 82, 84, 88, 98
– – pedicle of 74, 78, 82, 84, 88, 100
– zygomatic 2, 6, 8, 18, 20, 24
Areolae, gastric 212, 216
Artery (-ies)
– adrenal 250
– – inferior 250
– – middle 250
– – superior 250
– angular gyral 28
– appendicular 224
– arcuate 248
– basilar 40, 42
– brachial 114
– – muscular branches 114
– – profunda 114
– brachiocephalic. *See* Trunk
– calcarine 40
– callosomarginal 28, 30
– carotid
– – common
– – – left 174, 176, 180, 182
– – – right 174, 180, 182
– – external 182
– – internal 28, 30, 182
– cerebellar
– – inferior
– – – anterior 42
– – – posterior 40, 42
– – superior 40, 42
– cerebral
– – anterior 28, 30
– – middle 28, 30
– – posterior 40, 42
– cervical 182
– choroidal
– – anterior 28
– – posterior 40
– colic
– – left 226
– – middle 224
– – right 224
– collateral
– – radial 114
– – ulnar 114
– – – inferior 114
– – – superior 114
– communicating, posterior 40
– coronary 176, 184, 186, 188, 190
– – atrial branch
– – – posterior 186, 188
– – – middle 190

Artery, coronary
– – atrioventricular node branch 184
– – circumflex branch 188, 190
– – conus arteriosus branch 184, 188
– – diagonal branch 188, 190
– – interventricular branch
– – – anterior 188, 190
– – – posterior 184, 186, 188
– – marginal branch 184, 186, 188
– – posterolateral branch 184, 186, 188
– – septal branches 184, 188, 190
– – sinoatrial node branch 184
– – ventricular branch 186
– – – anterior 184, 188
– – – posterior 184, 188
– cystic 220
– digital, palmar
– – common 122
– – proper 122
– dorsalis pedis 148
– epigastric, inferior 106
– femoral 106, 138
– – deep 106
– frontopolar 28
– gastric
– – left 220, 250
– – right 220
– gastroduodenal 220, 250
– gastroepiploic
– – epiploic and gastric branches 220
– – left 220
– – right 220, 250
– genicular
– – descending 138
– – inferior, medial 138
– – middle 138
– – superior
– – – lateral 138
– – – medial 138
– gluteal, superior 106
– hepatic
– – common 220, 228, 250
– – left branch 220, 250
– – middle branch 220
– – proper 220, 228, 250
– – right branch 220, 250
– ileal 224, 250
– ileocolic 224, 250
– iliac
– – common 96, 98, 106, 226, 250
– – deep circumflex 106
– – external 106
– – internal 106
– – iliolumbar 106
– intercostal 180

Artery
- interlobar, of kidney 248
- interosseous
- – anterior 114, 122
- – common 114
- – posterior 114
- – recurrent 114
- jejunal 224, 250
- lenticular 30
- lumbar 106, 250
- malleolar, lateral anterior 148
- marginal, of colon 224
- mesenteric
- – inferior 226
- – superior 178, 224, 230, 250
- obturator 106
- occipital, lateral 42
- ophthalmic 28, 30
- pancreatic
- – branches 220
- – posterior 220
- pancreaticoduodenal
- – inferior 250
- – superior 220
- perforating 40
- pericallosal 28, 30, 42
- phrenic, inferior 250
- popliteal 138
- princeps pollicis 122
- pudendal, internal 106
- pulmonary (left or right) 150, 154, 176
- – basal part 150
- – branches to lobes 154, 172
- – intermediate part 150
- radial 114, 122
- – collateral 114
- – indicis 122
- – muscular branches 114
- – recurrent 114
- rectal, superior 226
- renal (left or right) 248, 250
- – anterior branch 248
- – capsular branch 248
- – posterior branch 248
- – ureteric branch 248
- sacral
- – lateral 106
- – medial 106, 250
- – segmental 248
- sigmoid 226
- splenic 220, 228, 250
- – pancreatic branches 220
- striate, anterior (Heubner) 30
- subcentral 28
- subclavian 174, 176, 178, 180, 182
- supramarginal 28
- temporal 28
- thoracic, internal 174, 180, 182
- thyroid, inferior 182
- tibial 138, 148
- – anterior 138, 148
- – posterior 138, 148
- ulnar 114, 122
- – collateral
- – – inferior 114
- – – superior 114
- – cutaneous branch 122

Artery, ulnar
- – deep palmar branch 122
- – recurrent 114
- uterine 106
- vertebral 42, 180, 182
- – muscular branches 40
Articulation(s)
- atlantoaxial
- – lateral 62, 64
- – median 66
- costotransversalis 82
- costovertebral 82
- intervertebral 62, 68, 70, 72, 74, 78, 82, 84, 96, 98
- vertebral lip 62
Atlas 14, 70, 72, 74
- arch of 2, 4, 6, 64, 68, 202
- posterior tubercle of 4
- transverse process of 2, 64
Atrium
- left 168, 170, 176, 178, 180, 204
- right 154, 166, 170, 172, 176, 178, 180
Auricle of atrium
- left 150, 166, 174
- right 176
Axis
- body of 64, 68, 70, 72, 74
- dens (odontoid process) of 2, 4, 6, 14, 20, 60, 62, 64, 66, 68
- spinous process of 4
- transverse process of 68

Barium sulfate, *XVI*
Bladder, urinary 102, 226, 246
Body
- adipose
- – of heart 166
- – of sole 146
- of axis 64, 68, 70, 72, 74
- of gall bladder 236, 238, 240
- of humerus 110, 178
- of hyoid bone 68
- of ischium 124, 126
- of lateral ventricle 48
- of mandible 18, 62, 64, 182
- of metacarpal bone 116
- pineal. *See* Gland
- of sternum 152, 186
- – ossification centers of 164
- of stomach 208, 210, 212
Bone(s)
- capitate 116, 118, 120
- cuboid 140, 142, 144, 146
- cuneiform
- – intermediate 142, 144, 146
- – lateral 142, 144, 146
- – medial 140, 142, 144, 146
- frontal
- – diploe of 4
- – external lamina of 4
- – internal lamina of 4
- – orbital part of 4
- hamate 116, 118, 120
- – hook 116
- hyoid 4, 70, 198, 202
- – body of 68
- lunate 116, 118, 120

Bone(s)
- metacarpal
- – 1st 116, 118, 120
- – 5th 116
- metatarsal 146
- – 1st 140, 144
- – 2nd 140
- – 5th 144
- nasal 4, 6, 16
- navicular 140, 142, 144, 146
- occipital 68, 70, 72, 74, 76
- petrous 24
- pisiform 116, 118, 120
- pubic 124. *See also* Pubis
- scaphoid 116, 118, 120
- sesamoid 116, 118, 120, 144, 146
- – of foot 144, 146
- – of hand 116, 118, 120
- sphenoid
- – greater wing 4, 12
- – lesser wing 16, 18, 20
- talonavicular 146
- temporal 20, 22, 68
- trapezium 116, 118, 120
- trapezoid 116, 120
- triquetral 116, 118, 120
- zygomatic 43
- *see also specific listings*
Branch, of pubis
- inferior 124
- superior 124
- *see also* Ramus
Breast 192, 194
- contour of 150, 208, 214
- nipple of 192, 194
Bronchus 78, 82, 166
- intermediate 156, 158
- lobar
- – inferior 152, 154, 156, 158, 160, 162
- – middle 154, 156, 158
- – superior 154, 156, 158, 160, 162, 170
- primary
- – left 82, 150, 152, 154, 160, 162, 168, 170, 204, 206
- – right 82, 150, 152, 154, 156, 158, 168, 170
- segmental
- – anterior 158, 160, 162
- – apical 156, 158, 160
- – apicoposterior 160, 162
- – basal 156, 158, 160, 162
- – lateral 156, 158
- – lingular 160, 162
- – posterior 158, 160, 162
- – superior 154, 156
- subsegmental, apical 162
Bulb
- aortic 174
- duodenal 208, 210, 228
- of internal jugular veins
- – inferior 172
- – superior 36
Bursa, suprapatellar 134

Calcaneus 142, 144, 146
- tuber of 142
Calvaria 18, 48

Calyces, renal 246, 248
Canal(s)
– cervical 274
– for diploic veins 4
– hypoglossal 12
– incisive 26
– infraorbital 18
– mandibular 26
– nasolacrimal 26
– optic 10, 20
– for pharyngotympanic tube 8
– of pulp 26
– pyloric 210, 212, 216
– sacral 104
– semicircular
– – anterior 20
– – lateral 20
– – posterior 24
Capitulum of humerus 112
Capsule, internal 54
Carina 150
Cartilage
– articular 134, 136
– cricoid
– – arch of 198
– – lamina of 68, 198
– thyroid 196
– – lamina of 62
Cauda equina 90, 92, 94, 96, 98, 100
Cavity
– articular 134, 136
– glenoid, of scapula 108, 110
– oral 4, 198, 202
– peritoneal 274
– of pulp 26
– of septum pellucidum 46
– tympanic 8, 22
– uterine 274
– see also Space
Cecum 234
Cells
– ethmoidal 2, 4, 6, 8, 12, 16, 18, 20
– mastoid 2, 6, 8, 10, 12, 20, 22, 24
– supraorbital 16
Cerebellum 52, 54
Cistern
– ambient 52, 54
– chiasmatic 52
– insula 54
– interpeduncular 52
– pontine 60
– quadrigeminal 52
Clavicle 62, 72, 80, 108, 110, 150, 152, 178, 180, 182, 196, 200, 204, 270
Clivus (Blumenbach) 4, 6, 12, 24, 28, 40
Coccyx 102, 104, 124, 232
Cochlea 24
Colliculi, midbrain 52, 60
Colon 102, 230, 254
– ascending 226, 234
– descending 226, 232, 234
– sigmoid 224, 226, 232, 234
– transverse 210, 234, 242
Commissure, posterior 50
Computed tomography.
    See Tomography

Concha, nasal
– inferior 2, 16, 18, 60
– medial 60
Condyle
– of femur
– – lateral 130, 132, 134, 136
– – medial 130, 132, 134, 136
– occipital 8
– of tibia
– – lateral 130
– – medial 130, 136
Confluence of sinuses 36, 38, 44, 58, 60
Constriction, peristaltic 212, 216
Contraction, peristaltic 208
Contrast media, XV–XVI
Conus arteriosus 168, 176
Cord, of spine. See Spinal cord
Corpus callosum
– rostrum of 60
– splenium of 60
– trunk of 46
Crest
– acetabular 124
– frontal, internal 2
– iliac 86, 88, 102, 104, 224, 236, 240, 250
– intertrochanteric 102, 124, 126, 268
– sacral, median 104
Crista galli 2, 4, 8, 18, 20
Cuneus 60
Curvature of stomach
– greater 208, 210, 212, 214, 216
– lesser 208, 210, 212, 214, 216

Dens (odontoid process) of axis 2, 4, 6, 14, 20, 60, 62, 64, 66, 68
Diaphragm 78, 150, 152, 164, 166, 170, 172, 174, 180, 184, 186, 188, 204, 206, 208, 210, 214, 222, 240, 244
– crus of 228, 230, 254
Diaphysis, femoral 128
Diploe, of frontal bone 4, 60
Disc, intervertebral 60, 70, 72, 86, 94, 98, 100
Dorsum sellae 4, 10, 50
Duct
– of caudate lobe
– – left 244
– – right 244
– common, bile 240, 242, 244
– cystic 238, 240, 242, 244
– hepatic
– – common 240, 242, 244
– – left 240, 242, 244
– – – lateral branch 244
– – right 240
– – – anterior branch 242, 244
– – – posterior branch 242, 244
– pancreatic 242, 244
– thoracic 272
Duodenum 208, 210, 216
– ascending part of 242
– descending part of 228, 230, 240, 242, 244, 254
– flexure of 210
– horizontal part of 242
Dural sac 90, 92, 94

Ear
– fetal 276
– outer 10, 12, 14, 22, 24
Eminence
– iliopubic 102
– intercondylar 132, 136
Epicondyle
– of femur
– – lateral 130
– – medial 130
– of humerus 112
Epiglottis 60, 200, 202
Epipharynx 202
Esophagus 154, 156, 158, 200, 202, 204, 206, 208
– abdominal part 214
– thoracic part 214
Eyeball 58
– lens 58

Falx cerebri 56
Fat, in breast 192
Femur 102, 132, 134, 138, 258
– condyle of
– – lateral 130, 132, 134, 136
– – medial 130, 132, 134, 136
– diaphysis of 128
– epicondyle of
– – lateral 130
– – medial 130
– fetal 276
– head of 102, 124, 126, 218, 232, 268
– – fovea of 102
– – ossification center in 128
– intercondylar eminence 132
– neck of 102, 124, 126
– shaft of 126
– tubercle of 130
Fetus, radiograph of 276
Fibula 132, 134, 138, 140, 142, 144, 146, 148
– fetal 276
– head of 130, 132
– shaft of 130
Fimbriae of uterine tube 274
Fissure
– cerebral 52, 54, 56, 58
– orbital
– – inferior 8
– – superior 2, 18
– – see also Rima
Flexure
– colic
– – left 224, 226, 234, 238, 254
– – right 224, 234, 236, 240
– duodenal
– – inferior 210
– – superior 210
– duodenojejunal 210, 242, 244
– hilum 150, 166
Fluoroscopy, equipment, XIII, XV
Folds
– aryepiglottic 202
– gastric 224
– mucosal, of stomach 212
– transverse rectal (Kohlrausch) 232

Foramen
- infraorbital 16
- intervertebral 74, 80, 82, 88, 94
- jugular 8, 12
- lacerum 8
- magnum 4, 6, 8, 12, 76
- mental 26
- obturator 102, 124, 126, 274
- ovale 6, 8, 12, 18
- rotundum 2, 18
- spinosum 6, 8, 12, 18
- stylomastoid 12
- transversarium 66
Fossa
- acetabular 102, 124, 126, 128
- articular, of temporal bone 22
- cerebral 54
- coronoid 112
- cranial, middle 6, 8, 12, 18, 50
- hypophyseal 2, 4, 10, 16, 18, 48, 50
- mandibular 20
- olecranon 112
- radial 112
- temporal 24
Fovea of head of femur 102.
  See also Pits
Fundus
- of gallbladder 236, 238, 240
- of stomach 150, 204, 206, 208, 210, 212, 214, 216, 222, 242
- of uterus 274

Gallbladder 228, 242
- body of 236, 238, 240
- fundus of 236, 238, 240
- neck of 236, 238, 240
Ganglion, spinal 82
Gases, for negative contrast media, *XVI*
Genu
- of corpus callosum 60
- of internal capsule 54
Gland
- adrenal 228, 230, 252, 254
- pineal 54
Groove(s)
- for middle meningeal artery 4, 18
- for sigmoid sinus 8, 22
- for sphenoparietal sinuses 4, 50
- for transverse sinus 8
Gyrus, cingulate 60

Head
- of caudate nucleus 46, 54
- of femur 102, 124, 126, 218, 232, 268
- - fovea of 102
- - ossification center in 128
- fetal 274
- of fibula 130, 132
- of humerus 108, 110, 178, 270
- of mandible 6, 12, 20, 22, 24, 50
- of radius 112
- of rib 78
- of talus 142, 144
Heart 78, 152, 164, 220, 244
- apex of 178
- *see also specific structures*
Hiatus, sacral 104

Hilus, renal 248
Hook of hamate bone 116
Horn
- of lateral cerebral ventricle
- - anterior 46, 48, 54, 58
- - inferior 48
- - occipital 58
- - posterior 48
- - sacral 104
Humerus 108, 110, 112, 152
- anatomical neck 108, 110
- body of 110, 178
- capitulum of 112
- epicondyle of 112
- fetal 276
- head of 108, 110, 178, 270
- neck of
- - anatomical 108, 110
- - surgical 108, 110
- trochlea of 112
- trochlear notch of 112
- tubercles of 108, 110
Hypopharynx 202
Hypophysis 60

Ileum 218
- terminal loop 234
Ilium
- ala of 102
- - fetal 276
- crest of 86, 88
- ossification center of 128
Image-intensifier television system, *XII–XIV*
Imaging techniques
- negative contrast media, *XVI–XVII*
- plain films, *XV*
- - attenuation effects, *XV*
- positive contrast media, *XVI*
Impression, gyral 12
Incus 24
Infundibulum
- of calyces 248
- of right ventricle (conus arteriosus) 176
Intestine
- fetal 276
- loops of 228, 230
Ischium
- body of 124, 126
- ossification center of 128
- spine of 102, 104, 124, 126, 274
- tuberosity of 102, 124, 126
Isthmus, of cervical canal of uterus 274

Jejunum 208, 210, 218, 242
Joint(s)
- acromioclavicular 108
- atlantoaxial, lateral 66, 220. *See also* Articulation
- ankle 140
- atlantooccipital 2
- calcaneocuboid 142, 144, 146
- interphalangeal
- - distal 116
- - proximal 116

Joint(s)
- metacarpophalangeal 116
- radioulnar
- - distal 116
- - proximal 112
- sacroiliac 88, 102, 124, 126, 218, 274
- subtalar 142
- talocalcaneonavicular 142
- talocrural 140, 142
- talonavicular 142
- temporomandibular 12, 24
Jugum cerebrale 12
Jugum, sphenoid 52

Kidney 88, 228, 230, 246, 252, 254
- calyces 246, 248
- hilus 248
- papilla 248
- pelvis 246, 248
- sinus 254
Kohler's anatomic teardrop 102, 124, 268

Labyrinth, bony 22
Labrum, acetabular 102. *See also* Lip
Lamina 82
- of cricoid cartilage 68, 198
- quadrigemina 52
- of skull bones
- - external 4, 60
- - internal 2, 4, 60
- of thyroid cartilage 62
- of vertebral arch 78, 88, 96, 98
Larynx 70
- ventricle of 198, 202
- vestibule of 196
Ligament
- medial collateral 136
- patellar 134
- suspensory, of mammary gland 192
Ligamentum flavum 96, 98, 100
Line
- Higenreiner's Y-symphyseal 128
- innominate 2, 16, 18
- Ombrédanne's vertical 128
- orbito-meatal 1
- paravertebral 78
- Shenton's 128
Linea terminalis 218
Lip
- of mouth 16, 60
- of vertebra, lateral 62
- *see also* Labrum
Liver 178, 220, 252
Lobe
- caudate 228, 230, 244, 254
- hepatic 228, 230, 254
- quadrate 228, 230
Lobulus
- postcentral 60
- precentral 60
Ludloff's spot 132

Malleolus
- lateral 140, 142, 144, 146
- medial 140, 142, 144
Malleus 24

Mandible 6, 60, 198, 200, 202
- body of 18, 62, 64, 182
- condylar process of 4, 6, 64, 68, 70, 72, 74
- coronoid process of 4, 6, 16, 18, 26, 64
- head of 6, 12, 20, 22, 24, 50
- ramus of 14, 26, 182
Manubrium, sternal 152, 164, 186
Margin
- acetabular 124, 128
- infraorbital 16, 18, 26
- medial, of scapula 150
- orbital 4
- supraorbital 2, 18, 20
- see also Crest, Ridge(s)
Maxilla
- alveolar process of 14, 16
- lateral contour 2
- zygomatic process of 4
Meatus, acoustic
- external 4, 12, 22, 24
- internal 6, 8, 10, 20, 22, 24
Medulla oblongata 60
Membrane
- tectorial, inferior, of L4, 98
- tympanic 12, 24
Meniscus, medial 136
Mesencephalon 58
Muscle
- buccalis 14
- erector spinae 228, 230
- masseter 14
psoas major 88, 96, 98, 230, 240, 246, 252
- pterygoid, medial 14
- rectus
- - lateral 58
- - medial 58
- scalene, anterior 78
Musculature, cervical 14
Myocardium, left ventricular 174

Nasopharynx 14, 60, 202
Neck
- of femur 102, 124, 126
- of gallbladder 236, 238, 240
- of humerus
- - anatomical 108, 110
- - surgical 108, 110
- of radius 112
- of rib 78
- of talus 142
Nerve(s)
- facial 24
- optic 58
- spinal 90, 96
- vestibulocochlear 24
Nipple 192, 194
Nodes, lymph
- axillary 270
- brachial 270
- iliac
- - common 260, 262, 264, 266
- - external 260, 262, 266
- - internal 260, 262, 266
- infraclavicular 270
- inguinal

Nodes, lymph, inguinal
- - deep 268
- - superficial 260, 266
- paraaortic 262, 264, 266
- pectoral 270
- supraclavicular 270
Nose 60
Notch
- angular, of stomach 212, 216
- cardiac 208
- interarytenoid 200
- scapular 110
- sciatic
- - greater 102, 104, 124
- - lesser 104
- trochlear (semilunar), of humerus 112
- ulnar 116
Nucleus
- caudate, head of 46, 54
- lenticular 54

Obturator foramen 102, 124, 126, 274
- exotosis of 124
Olecranon 112
Orbit 12, 16, 18, 20
- margin of 4
- - infraorbital 16, 18, 26
- - supraorbital 2, 18, 20
- roof of 2, 18, 20
- wall of
- - lateral 6, 8
- - medial 2
Orifice, uterine, of uterine tube 274
Ossification center(s)
- of femur 128
- of ilium 128
- of ischium 128
- of pubis 128
- of sternum 164

Palate
- hard 4, 26, 60
- soft 4, 198
Pancreas 228, 230, 254
- uncinate process of 230
Papilla
- duodenal, greater (Vater) 244
- renal 248
Parenchyma, glandular 194
Patella 130, 132, 134, 136, 138
- articulation facets of 136
Pecten of pubis 102
Pelvis, renal 220, 226, 246, 248, 264
Pedicle, of vertebral arch 74, 78, 82, 84, 88, 100
Phalanx
- base of 116
- distal 116, 144
- head of 116
- middle 116, 144
- proximal 116, 144
Pharynx 4, 6, 66, 68, 70, 72, 74, 200
- laryngeal 62, 196
- nasal part of 4
- oral 202
- piriform recess of 196, 200, 202

Pits, granular 2
Plane
- nuchal 2, 16, 64
- sphenoid 2, 4, 10, 16, 18, 20, 50
Plate
- cribriform 4
- quadrigeminal 60
Pleura, mediastinal 154
Plexus
- choroid, of lateral cerebral ventricle 54
- venous, anterior vertebral 96
Pons 24, 60
Popliteal surface 132
Porta hepatis 228
Precuneus 60
Process
- alveolar, of maxilla 14, 16
- articular, of vertebrae 82
- - inferior 68, 74, 78, 84, 86, 88, 96, 98
- - superior 68, 74, 78, 84, 86, 88, 96, 98
- clinoid
- - anterior 4, 8, 10, 50
- - posterior 4, 10, 50
- condylar, of mandible 4, 6, 64, 68, 70, 72, 74
- coracoid 108, 110, 270
- coronoid
- - of mandible 4, 6, 16, 18, 26, 64
- - of ulna 112
- costal 84, 86, 88
- frontal, of zygomatic bone 4
- mastoid 2, 14, 20, 22, 74
- odentoid, of axis. See Dens
- posterior, of talus 142, 146
- pterygoid 6, 8, 14, 18
- of rib 100
- spinous 62, 64, 66, 68, 74, 78, 82, 84, 88, 96, 98, 104
- - of axis 4
- - of C7, 80
- - of L2, 86
- - of T1, 78, 80
- styloid
- - of radius 116, 118
- - of temporal bone 2, 14, 22, 64, 66
- - of ulna 116, 118, 120
- temporal, of zygomatic bone 26
- transverse
- - of atlas 2, 64, 66
- - of axis 68
- - of vertebrae 62, 78, 82
- uncinate, of pancreas 230
- ungulate 116
- zygomatic, of maxilla 4, 12, 22
Promontory of sacrum 86, 104, 232
Protuberance
- mental 2, 4, 26, 64
- occipital, internal 54
Pubis
- branch (or ramus) of
- - inferior 102, 124
- - superior 102, 124
- ossification center of 128
- pecten of 102
- symphysis of 102, 124, 234
Pulp, of tooth 26
Pylorus 208, 210

Pylorus
– muscular sphincter of 216
Pyramid, petrous 22
– apex of 20

Radiation
– absorbed, *XI*
– ionizing, *XI*
– units of energy, *XI*
Radiographic equipment, *XI–XIII*
– focusing grid, *XII*
– intensifier screen, *XII*
– magnification and sharpness, *XII*
Radiographs. *See* X-rays
Radiography, cassetteless, *XII*
Radiology, diagnostic, physical units, *XI*
Radius 112, 116, 118, 120
– fetal 276
– head of 112
– neck of 112
– styloid process of 116, 118
Ramus
– of mandible 14, 26, 182
– of pubis
– – inferior 102
– – superior 102
– – *see also* Branch
Recess
– costodiaphragmatic 150
– infundibular 50
– optic 50
– periradicular 90
– pineal 50
– piriform 196, 200, 202
– suprapineal 50
Rectum 232, 234
– ampulla of 232
– transverse fold of 232
Rib 82
– 1st 62, 74, 78, 80, 150, 172, 200
– 2nd 80, 108
– 11th 86, 88, 238, 244, 246
– 12th 86, 88, 214, 238, 240, 248
– – process of 100
– fetal 276
Ridge(s)
– longitudinal, of stomach 212, 214, 216
– occipital, internal 20
– petrous 2, 4, 16, 18, 20, 22, 50
– *see also* Crest, Margin
Rima glottidis 196
Roentgen, William Conrad, *X*
Root, spinal 76, 92

Sacrum 86, 94, 102, 104, 124, 232, 274
Scapula 78, 178, 270
– angle of
– – inferior 108
– – superior 62, 108, 150, 196
– border of
– – lateral 108
– – medial 108
– coracoid process of 108, 110
– fetal 276
– glenoid cavity of 108, 110
– margin of, medial 150
– notch of 110

Scapula
– spine of 108, 110
Seldinger technique, *XVI*
Sella turcica 22, 50
Septum(-a)
– interalveolar 26
– interventricular 178
– nasal 2, 6, 8, 16, 18, 26
– pellucidum 46, 54, 60
Shaft
– of femur 126
– of fibula 130
– of tibia 130
– *see also* Body
Shoulder 68
Sinus(-es)
– aortic (Valsalva) 176, 190
– confluence of 36, 38, 44, 58, 60
– frontal 2, 4, 10, 12, 16, 18, 20, 46
– maxillary 2, 4, 6, 8, 16, 18, 20, 24, 26
– occipital 36, 38
– paranasal 18
– renal 230, 254
– sagittal, superior 32, 34, 36, 38, 44, 56, 60
– sigmoid 4, 8, 36, 38
– sphenoid 4, 6, 8, 12, 16, 18, 20, 22, 24, 50, 60
– sphenoparietal 4, 10, 36, 50
– straight 34, 44
– tarsal 142
– transverse 20, 36, 38
– – groove for 8
– of venous valve 258
Skin 60
Space
– intervertebral 72, 86
– retrocardiac 164
– retrocrural 230, 254
– retrosternal 164
– subarachnoid 76, 90, 92
– *see also* Cavity
Sphincter, esophageal 202
Spinal cord 60, 66, 82
– root 76, 92
Spine
– iliac
– – anterior
– – – inferior 102, 124, 126
– – – superior 102, 124, 126
– – posterior
– – – inferior 102
– – – superior 102
– ischial 102, 104, 124, 126, 274
– nasal
– – anterior 4, 26
– – posterior 4, 6, 8
– of scapula 108, 110
Spleen 220, 222, 228, 230, 254
– accessory 254
Squamous suture 10
Sternum 178
– angle of 152, 186
– body of 152, 186
– – ossification centers of 164
Stomach 78, 208, 210, 224

Stomach
– body of 208, 210, 212
– cardiac portion of 214
– constriction of, peristaltic 212, 216
– curvature of
– – greater 208, 210, 212, 214, 216
– – lesser 208, 210, 212, 214, 216
– folds of, mucosal 212
– fundus of 150, 204, 206, 208, 210, 212, 214, 216, 222, 242
– notch of, angular 212, 216
– pyloric part of 228, 230
Substance
– gray 54, 56
– white 54, 56
Sulcus
– calcerine 60
– central 60
– cingulate 60
– parietooccipital 60
– *see also* Groove
Suture
– coronal 4
– frontozygomatic 2, 4, 26
– intermaxillary 26
– lambdoid 2, 4, 10
– occipitomastoid 22
– sagittal 2, 8, 18
– squamous 10
– temporozygomatic 26
Symphysis
– of pubis 102, 124, 234
– Y- 128

Talus 142, 146, 148
– head of 142, 144
– neck 142
– posterior process of 142, 146
– trochlea 140, 142
Teeth
– canine 26
– foramen at apex of 26
– incisive 26
– molar 26
– premolar 26
– pulp
– – canal 26
– – cavity 26
Thalamus 54, 60
Thymus 164
Tibia 134, 138, 140, 142, 144, 146, 148
– condyle of
– – lateral 130
– – medial 130, 136
– fetal 276
– eminence of, intercondylar 136
– shaft of 130
– tubercle of, intercondylar 130
– tuberosity of 132
Tissue
– parenchymal 192
– periductal 192
– subcutaneous, of skull 60
Tomography
– computed, *XIII*
– transverse axial, *XIII*
Tongue 60, 68, 202

Torcular Herophili. *See* Confluence, Sinus
Trachea 62, 68, 70, 74, 78, 80, 82, 150,
    152, 154, 156, 164, 168, 170, 196, 198,
    200, 202, 206
– bifurcation of 150, 154
Tragus 10
Trochanter
– greater 102, 124, 126
– lesser 102, 124, 126, 260, 268
Trochlea
– of humerus 112
– of talus 140, 142
Trunk
– brachiocephalic 176, 178, 180,
    182
– bronchomediastinal 272
– celiac 178, 220, 222, 228, 250, 254
– jugular 272
– pulmonary 150, 154, 166, 168, 174, 176,
    178
– subclavian 272
– thyrocervical 182
Tube, uterine 274
Tuber of calcaneus 142
Tubercle
– adductor, of femur 130
– of anterior scalene muscle 78
– articular, of temporal bone 22, 68
– of atlas
– – anterior 66
– – posterior 4
– of humerus
– – greater 108, 110
– – lesser 108, 110
– infraglenoid 270
– pubic 124
– of rib 62, 78, 196
– of tibia, intercondylar
– – lateral 130
– – medial 130
– pubic 124
Tuberculum sellae 4, 50
Tuberosity
– ischial 102, 124, 126
– of distal phalanx (hand) 116
– of metatarsal bone 142, 144,
    146
– radial 112
– of scaphoid bone 118
– of tibia 132

Ulna 112, 116, 118, 120
– coronoid process of 112
– fetal 276
– styloid process of 116, 118, 120
Ureter 220, 226, 246, 248, 264
Uterus 106, 274
– cervical canal of 274
– fundus of 274
Uvula
– of cerebellum 60
– of palate 60, 202

Vallecula, epiglottic 200, 202
Valves
– aortic 180
– venous 256, 258
Vein(s)
– adrenal 230
– anastomotic 32, 34, 36
– – inferior (Labbé) 34
– – superior (Trolard) 32, 34, 36
– axillary 172
– azygos 154, 172, 176, 228
– basal (Rosenthal) 44
– brachiocephalic 172, 174
– caval. *See subentry* vena cava
– cephalic 172
– cerebellar 36, 38
– cerebral
– – great (Galen) 44
– – internal 44
– – superficial middle 34
– – superior 32, 34, 36, 38, 44
– choroid 44
– communicating (lower leg) 256
– deep (of lower leg) 256
– diploic 48
– hemiazygos 228
– jugular
– – external 172
– – internal 172, 174
– – – bulbs of 36, 172
– lumbar 96
– mesenteric
– – inferior 228
– – superior 230
– pontine, middle 44
– popliteal 256
– portal 222, 228, 230
– pulmonary 150, 152, 154, 166
– – inferior
– – – left 176
– – – right 174, 176
– – superior
– – – left 174, 176
– – – right 174, 176
– renal 230
– saphenous
– – great 256, 258
– – small 256
– splenic 222, 228, 230
– subclavian 172, 174
– subcutaneous 256
– testicular 230
– thyroid ima 172
– vena cava
– – inferior 96, 98, 150, 166, 228, 230, 254
– – superior 150, 154, 166, 172, 174, 176,
    178, 180
Ventricle
– of cerebrum
– – fourth 50, 54, 60
– – lateral
– – – anterior horn of 46, 48, 54, 58

Ventricle of cerebrum, lateral
– – – body of 48
– – – central portion of 56
– – – choroid plexus of 54
– – – inferior horn of 48
– – – occipital horn of 58
– – – posterior horn of 48
– – third 48, 50, 54
– of heart
– – left 150, 154, 166, 168, 170, 172, 174,
    176, 178
– – right 170, 172, 176, 178
– of larynx 198, 202
Vermis, cerebellar 52, 54, 58, 60
Vertebrae
– cervical 6, 62
– – C3, 68, 70, 72, 198
– – C4, 60, 74
– – C7, 6, 80
– – enlargement 76
– fetal 276
– lumbar
– – L1, 210, 248, 252
– – L2, 222, 236, 238
– – L3, 84, 90, 94, 218, 246
– – L4, 88, 96, 102, 106, 234
– – L5, 92, 104, 232, 264
– prominens 68
– sacral 128
– – S1, 94
– – S2, 94
– thoracic
– – T1, 62, 78, 80
– – T4, 82
– – T6, 80
– – T7, 78
– – T10, 220
– – T11, 240, 244, 250
– – T12, 78, 172, 224, 242
Vermis, cerebellar 52, 54, 56, 60
Vessels
– lymphatic
– – afferent 268
– – efferent 268
– pulmonary 188, 190
Vestibule 20, 24
– of larynx 196
– of internal ear 20, 24
Vomer 4, 16

Wing of sphenoid bone
– greater 4, 12
– lesser 2, 16, 18, 20
– *see also* Ala

X-radiation, *XI*
X-ray television equipment, *XIII–XIV*
X-rays, directions of beam 1

Y-symphysis 128

Zonography, *XIII*